The
Teeth
Whitening
Cure

The Perfect Cure
for Bleach Fever

The Teeth Whitening Cure

A HOLISTIC GUIDE TO BRIGHT SMILES AND BETTER HEALTH IN A TOXIC WORLD

LESTER SAWICKI, D.D.S.

The Teeth Whitening Cure

http://www.revolutiontooth.com/

The author wishes to thank Ms. Li Zhang, the artist who produced
all of the brilliant custom graphics you'll find throughout this book...
George Foster the cover designer for it... William Groetzinger
its interior designer... and Edward and Lynne Green for its
proofreading/editing.

Library of Congress Control Number: 2009913935
ISBN: 0984370617
EAN: 9780984370610

I dedicate this book to
my sister Mrs. Lila Kasper,
my good friend Steve Shyman, and
my Doctor Don. X. Zhang DAOM, Ph.D. L.Ac.,
for sustaining my life in special and
loving ways I will never forget.

Contents

Preface

Our sun is the "Great Purifier." Its ionizing rays produce hydrogen peroxide (H_2O_2) in the atmosphere that helps cleanse the air of pollutants. Likewise, when we inhale nebulized hydrogen peroxide mist, the H_2O_2 cleanses our lungs, sinuses, throat, bronchial tract—areas most affected by viruses—by killing infected cells that are functioning as viral laboratory workshops. When used correctly, this natural therapeutic weapon of mass destruction cannot fail to wipe out all types of viral infections, and it does so without side effects. This "great purifier" burns away many toxic substances found on the internal and external surfaces of our bodies. We need only discover and unleash the science behind nature's cure for disease.

In my teeth whitening system, hydrogen peroxide is the chemical that bleaches stains out of teeth. I believe the safe, healthy use of hydrogen peroxide can not only whiten teeth, but also detoxify the body of impurities. In fact, it was a team of periodontists working to cure gum disease who discovered the teeth whitening "side-effect" of hydrogen peroxide.

However, teeth whitening is not a modern discovery. It was practiced in Greece and India for thousands of years. The ancient Greeks used urine to whiten their teeth and drank it as a remedy to cure disease, and ancient Ayurvedic texts from India reveal urine therapy to be one of their most powerful medicinal treatments for many types of disease. According to some sources, it may well be the most researched and most medically proven natural remedy.

Fortunately it is not necessary to drink urine in order to receive its health-promoting components as they are easily absorbed into the highly vascular oral mucosa when just rinsing with it. While rinsing, urea travels through oral tissues into the body's circulatory network and thereby exerts its holistic, disease-curing effect.

Hydrogen peroxide, either used for teeth whitening or as an internal detoxing cure, works similarly to urine—only better. And which internal diseases does hydrogen peroxide address? Most probably the same ones addressed by urine, and possibly more. Urea hydrogen peroxide was actually an ingredient in the prototypical teeth whitening gels, but the average consumer was unaware that they were rinsing with urea. I think most people would agree—and trust me, I know from personal experience—that the modern, flavored bleaching gels are preferable to urine.

Unfortunately there are problems with the manner in which teeth whitening systems are used today. This book fully addresses the issue of toxic dental bleaching gels and whitening products: teeth whitening, disease prevention and whole-body detoxification are the three main issues covered in this text, and together they constitute a complete system for better health.

Did you know that your teeth may act as a trap for toxic chemicals, drug-resistant bacteria, virulent viruses and hazardous radioactive isotopes, and that the tooth's circulatory system provides access to all of the body's vital organs? Any noxious substance absorbed into tooth enamel and dentin has the potential to end up in the heart, liver, kidneys, etc.

Preface

What happens if your dentist unintentionally locks these poisons into the complex labyrinth of the tooth's structure when cosmetically covering teeth with white fillings, veneers, or crowns? A frail tooth in a weakened immune system is a prime target for infestation. These are some of the many questions answered and issues illuminated in this breakthrough book.

Do you want a stunning, bright smile AND superior, overall health? I believe the two are mutually supportive, a yin and yang of natural beauty and a vibrant, healthy, long life. I hope you find this book informative, entertaining, and amazing—and perhaps a little shocking as well.

To your health,

Lester Sawicki, D.D.S.

The Teeth Whitening Cure

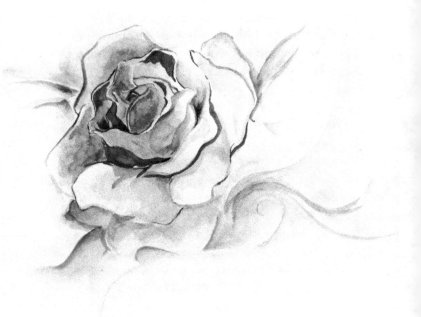

PROLOGUE

Do you want to heal and recover from disease and illness? Would you like to live a long, happy, healthy, prosperous life? At age 120 would you like to wake up in the morning after a deep, long, satisfying sleep, stretch nimbly as a cat, roar like a lion, and then fully pour your heart into another purpose driven day... The RICHEST, and BEST day of your life? Do you want super health and vitality?

It is my sincere hope this book will help people wake up into the practical reality of using a safe, natural, teeth whitening detox, as one means to the very real possibility of living fit and free 120 years and beyond.

Yes! I believe this is all possible and much of my belief stems from my own experience, observations, and research. Science has shown that the human body should have a normal life span of at least 120 years. "Normal" means healthy, fully functioning, and free of disease. This book will help people wake up into the practical reality of living fit and free 120 years and beyond. The knowledge assembled in this book will provide you with the necessary information to make the decision to either improve your health or continue to foster disease.

As a practicing dentist for thirty-three years, I've detailed for you exactly what steps must be taken to *revitalize the essential life force of your teeth.* I call it the "teeth detox". One surprising benefit is that you will also safely restore a genuinely whiter and gorgeous smile with a home whitening treatment costing only pennies a day (instead of the hundreds of dollars you'd pay to have it *professionally* done).

You see... I firmly believe the human body is capable of curing itself of any disease using mind, air, water, and food. The cure for all disease begins with your intentions. If you slip into disease and illness, then the best medicine is organic food found at your local supermarket. Yes, food is your best medicine: Organic vegetables, fruit, meat, fish, fowl, seeds, nuts, grains, herbs, and supplements. Fresh clean air and water are the necessary solvents and carriers of this nutrition to feed your body.

The cure for disease will never be found in a laboratory. I do believe, however, that God has given us the gift of western medical science to help us temporarily treat the uncomfortable symptoms of the diseases we have created. Once the body becomes more comfortable, we can easily cure it using natural means expressed through the wisdom of the ages.

Unfortunately we have been programmed to view aging negatively, and to believe there is nothing to be done other than accept physical and mental deterioration. Sadly, this negative and destructive thinking is a self-fulfilling prophecy. Science today has proven that your body reflects your beliefs. Mark my words... you will soon see hundreds of thousands of people living vibrant, youthful lives beyond the age of 120 due to their conscious choice to believe in positive expectations. It is my sincere desire that the information in this book can help you to begin the process of choosing and using positive beliefs and expectations in order to achieve and maintain perfect health.

Prologue

Three things must be accomplished if we expect to cure ourselves of any disease: we must hydrate, alkalize, and detoxify the body. There are many books available that teach you how to hydrate, alkalize, and detoxify the body. This book, "The Teeth Whitening Cure," is the only book you will find that explains in detail how you can help detoxify your body through the process of detoxifying and whitening your teeth.

As a dentist I can tell a lot about a person's health simply by looking at the condition of his or her mouth. Bad breath, tartar, plaque, swelling, inflammation, discoloration, staining, and other symptoms are signs of poor health. The mouth is not isolated. What happens inside the mouth reflects what is going on in other organs. I can spot signs of cancer, diabetes, gastrointestinal disorders, autoimmune disease, heavy metal contamination, heart disease, drug and alcohol abuse, and more.

The mouth not only reveals clues to the nature of the inside of the body, but it can also have direct influences on it. Oral infections such as gum disease, root canal infections, and tooth decay can cause any number of health problems. The discovery of the connection between oral health and the rest of the body dates back thousands of years and is recorded in Far Eastern medicine of China, India, and Tibet. It is also evident in Western medicine as far back as ancient Egypt, Greece, and Mesopotamia. For centuries the relationship between oral health and systemic health was considered so obvious that before livestock or slaves were purchased, the mouths of the livestock or slaves were examined by prospective purchasers.

Oral health can also affect the health of our unborn children. It helps lay the foundation for the health of our growing children all the way through adulthood. Oral bacteria, fungus, parasites, and viruses are released from the mother's saliva into her blood stream and then transferred to the developing embryo possibly causing low-grade inflammation that affects the mind as well as negatively influence systemic conditions.

The U.S. Department of Health and Human Services issued a detailed report from the Surgeon General clearly outlining and documenting the connection between oral health and systemic disease. When you read this report, you will be convinced that if you want to live 120 super-healthy, youthful years, then you must pay attention to your teeth. Your body was made to live at least 120 years and your teeth were made to last a lifetime—if you take care of them.

During my thirty-three years of dental practice, I have examined and interviewed a number of patients between 85 and 100 years old. I was amazed by their grace, agility, mental acuity, vitality, enthusiasm, and overall health. The healthiest among them had managed to retain most of their teeth through superior oral health care practices. This convinces me... there is a definite connection between good oral health and a healthy long life.

The discoveries in my dental practice and my own practical experiences help illuminate this book with thousands of years of wisdom from the East, PLUS the latest scientific discoveries of the West. These personal observations and discoveries—in concert with the ancient wisdom of the East and the most modern western research—led me to the conclusions which made this book possible. What I discovered is that the teeth and tongue comprise the main gateway into the body. They are perhaps the most important elements for overall health. They tear, grind, and chew the food, preparing it for the digestive tract, where, upon further reduction, all of the useful nutrition is transported through the blood stream and into our cells. What most amazed me is that teeth also absorb and excrete toxic waste. In fact, your whole body, including your teeth, is like a sponge. When functioning properly, nourishment is taken in and waste is excreted. When disease and illness occur... the system malfunctions and the results can be very 'ugly.'

Yes, I have discovered that there are good, bad, and ugly components to teeth. The good and bad components are normal. In a perfect world, the teeth absorb good and excrete bad. If this process is impeded, the result is 'ugly'. In very simple terms, if your teeth are stained, then your naturally balanced exchange of 'in with the good' and 'out with the bad' has been compromised. This disruption of natural flow affects every organ in your body in a negative way, possibly shortening your life span.

The good news is that to extend and improve your quality of life, you do not have to be in good health already. Don't worry about the past. What you do from this moment forward is what counts. You can begin to positively affect your overall health and longevity right now by improving your oral health.

Of course, a single book is not enough to chart a path to perfect health. THIS book, however, is the only source that reveals the secrets to "teeth detox" and how it relates to a healthier body.

It is my sincere wish what you're about to read here will enable you to become free to accept all of the good that life has to offer you, and you'll take advantage of your positive thoughts, beliefs, expectations, and imagination to make it happen for you.

As you pause for just a bit and consider what you've just read, let me tell you how this book has been structured for you to provide you 'options' you can use to suit your own reading style.

To combat the rather technical nature of many of the paragraphs I've created a 'little story' for those of you whose natures are more 'in tune' with this type of presentation. You'll want to continue directly onward, beginning the first of Chapter 1, where you'll meet Gayla Brighte-Smythe, and her family. She'll be the "author" who'll guide you humorously through your book purchase.

She will introduce you to her dentist friend, Dr. Q., who will enlighten you with the very important information I've accumulated on this subject during my thirty-three years in dental practice and will give you 'tips' enabling you to learn quickly all you ever wanted to know about HEALTHFUL teeth whitening... and MORE. Everything you'll read here comes from my own very extensive research and deeply held beliefs. And you can be assured I DO follow my own advice.

Lester Sawicki, DDS

Prologue

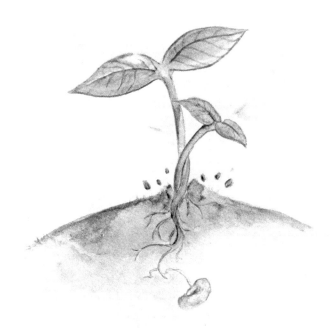

Chapter 1

The Ultimate Teeth Bleaching Treatment

Welcome!

and thank you...

...for spending a few minutes with me to learn what I consider the Ultimate Teeth Bleaching Treatment.

My name is Gayla Brighte-Smythe. I'm a 38 year old wife, mother of 3 gorgeous girls and 2 handsome boys, plus CEO of my own International Organic Confectionery Company. I'm also a self made millionaire who relies on my husband, Jake, to manage the household when I'm away on business trips.

It was spring break of the year 2009 when I decided to take my 5 adorable young adults on a business trip with me. Jake stayed behind in the United States golfing with friends. I was negotiating a deal with organic cacao farmers in Ecuador and wanted to spend a little quality time with the kids. We arranged a mini surfing tour of Ecuador's Pacific coastal beaches.

Ecuador straddles the equator and is bordered by Colombia on the north, Peru on the east and south, and the Pacific Ocean to the west. I convinced the kids that Ecuador is a world full of contrasts and marvels, great beaches, and breaks that would give them the most complete surf vacation one could ask for. With the surprise, adventure, beauty, nature, and incredible surf this promised them, they were sold!

My confectionery company specializes in food products made from the cacao bean. We are 100% organic and supply whole cacao beans, nibs, powder, and chocolate treats. All chocolate comes from the cacao bean, and I buy only Quality Raw, Unfermented, Certified Organic Cacao Beans from indigenous farmers in Ecuador. To ensure quality, we generally pay each farmer 25% more than the price for regular, organic cacao in Ecuador.

I have yet to come across a child (or for that matter an adult), who does not like chocolate. The main attraction in chocolates is in the "melt in mouth feeling" that comes from its low melting temperature. The well-known Ecuadorian cocoa of "delicate aroma," in fact, belongs to the Ecuadorian humid forest where cacao is farmed. The Maya and Aztec empires discovered the tasty secret of the cacao tree 2000 years ago.

Cacao has an extremely high energy content. It has historically been used as energy food, because it contains an ideal mix of fats, sugars, carbohydrates, and protein. It also contains high levels of catechin, fiber, B vitamins, and anti-oxidant-like substances. Calcium, Phosphates, and Vitamins A, C, and D occur in smaller quantities.

Cacao contains the same antioxidants (phenols) as red wine, which has been shown possibly to protect against heart disease. Pure dark Chocolate bars contain greater quantities than wine! The seeds are 54% cocoa butter, and, like olive oil and avocado, they do not raise blood cholesterol levels.

and...

Cacao, cocoa, and chocolate...

STAIN TEETH BROWN!!!

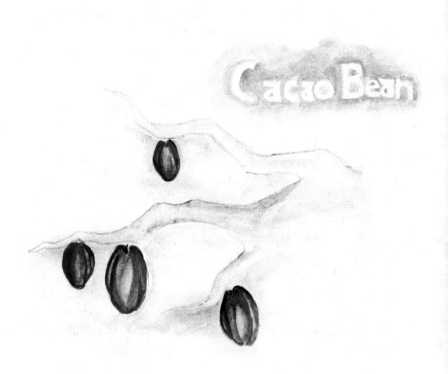

Chapter 2

Shocked and Delighted!

Yes, I have money, and plenty of it. My passion is chocolate, and I turned my passion into a very successful and rewarding business. My family shares in my passion quite willingly. We live, love, eat, drink, breathe, dance, dream, and sleep cacao. But cacao stains teeth brown, and... as a result, we are constantly struggling to keep our teeth white.

The 5 children, ages 14 to 22, are some of the healthiest kids you can imagine. I weaned them on cacao beans, nibs, powder, butter, and chocolate treats. I believe cacao is one of the healthiest energy foods on the planet, and I made certain it was a staple of their diet. They have explosive energy and unbreakable health. They also have brown stained teeth, just like their mom and dad.

My kids love chocolate, AND they want white teeth. Just before we left for Ecuador we visited our family dentist for our yearly check up. I inquired about teeth whitening and was shocked when the total cost to whiten teeth for all seven of us was quoted as $5600. THAT equates to $800 per mouth!

Admittedly, I have more than enough money, but I accumulated wealth through sweat, tears, and tough, scrappy, investment strategies. Saving money was the foundation of my success, and paying $5600 to whiten our teeth did not seem like a good investment... especially considering the results are ONLY temporary, not permanent.

I was also worried about the SAFETY of teeth bleaching. There were a number of recent news stories warning about the dangers of bleaching teeth. My dentist did not address safety issues to my satisfaction so I decided to give serious thought about professional teeth whitening during my business trip/surfing vacation.

In general, we are a healthy, loving, family, and I attribute much of this to well nourished mental and emotional development. I firmly believe that food plays an important role in my family's strong mind and spirit. That is why we are devout food purists. Only, and mostly raw, organic foods touch our palate. Organic cacao is a basic ingredient in our nutritional support.

I have already mentioned the high antioxidant properties of cacao, and eating chocolate causes the brain to produce natural opiates, which dull pain and

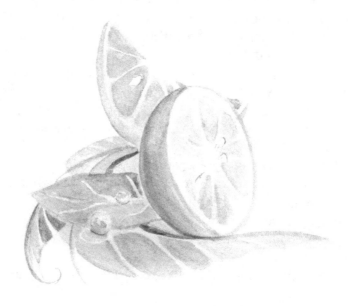

increase a feeling of wellbeing. The natural chemical in cacao, theobromide, is proven to cause both physical and mental relaxation, a sense of well-being and alertness. Chocolate is a "treat", something most people enjoy and cherish. This feeling has aphrodisiac effects, and for many centuries chocolate has been identified with love, and yes, with sex. This might explain why my family is so well balanced, energized, yet mellow. It also might shine light on why I have had 5 children with my husband, Jake.

But… cacao, and its food products, stain teeth brown, and this has recently become a family issue.

As my story continues, I was shocked and delighted to discover in Ecuador…

THE MOST POWERFUL AND ONLY
PRACTICAL ADVICE AVAILABLE…
…ON TEETH WHITENING.

Chapter 3

"Drowning in Teeth Bleach?"

I was on the sunny warm beach enjoying a Jugo natural—freshly squeezed juice called Naranjilla. This bitter orange fruit is too sour to eat in its solid form, but the thick green juice is delicious.

The boys and girls were surfing in the playful Pacific when all of a sudden Braen, my 17 year old, disappeared into the water with an echo of a desperate shout for help. Frightened, I dropped my Jugo and ran 75 yards to the water's edge. Two heads bobbed in the water as a rescuer guided Braen back to shore.

Braen, shaken and exhausted, trudged out of the water apparently safe. I held him in my arms praying

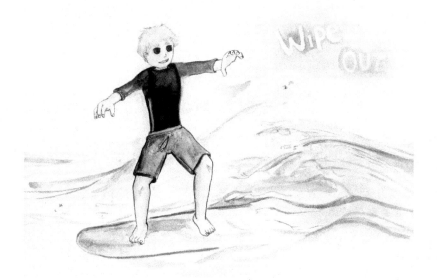

to God joyful praise. After a minute, I regained my composure and could not express in words my deep thanks to the rescuer. She smiled and humbly said it was nothing. I insisted that she have dinner with us and she accepted.

That evening we all met for dinner, and to my shock and delight Braen's rescuer was a dentist from New York. For the last 25 years she had been a Cosmetic Dentist to famous models, actors, politicians, and business moguls. She was now semi-retired and spending a little down time at her second home near Vilcacamba, a sleepy village in southern Ecuador. Vilcacamba is a subtropical place with lots of orange trees, nature preserves, waterfalls, and one of those regions you can consider rural. The area has been referred to as the "Playground of the Inca," which refers to its historic use as a retreat for Incan royalty.

Before and during dinner, we exchanged introductions and shared friendly conversation about our life in the States, as well as what we were doing in Ecuador. When dessert was being served... the children bridged in questions about whitening their brown teeth. This point in time became an epic moment in my family's life. We sat with jaws dropped as we listened to our guest give us a brief treatise on the subject.

Her first words were...

"MODERN DENTISTRY IS DEAD WRONG"

"Braen, remember the feeling you had when you were fighting for your life today? You were drowning in the waters of the Pacific, and I'm sure you will have

nightmares over the incident. I'm about to make a statement which may surprise you but,

**Americans are Drowning
in a Sea of Toxic Teeth Bleach.**"

We all had puzzled expressions on our tired faces, and dessert was over. Our new friend's body language indicated it was time to say good-byes. Everyone looked forward to a restful night of sleep. She did, however, leave her e-mail address, and graciously advised us she would be glad to answer all our e-mailed questions to her about teeth whitening.

That night in bed I drifted into sleep with our friend's words on my mind...

"MODERN DENTISTRY IS DEAD WRONG...
DROWNING IN TEETH BLEACH."

Chapter 4

Modern Dentistry is Dead Wrong

We reluctantly ended our Ecuador adventure, the
children returned to school, and I resumed business as
usual. Braen, however, was emotionally bonded to his
rescuer. At his age it is normal to develop a bond very
quickly under emotional stress. During the first few
weeks after our return, he would often exclaim, *"her
teeth were so-o-o white! I wish I had her bright smile!
She could sure flash 'em!"*

I decided it might be good experience, and an education for him to contact his Cosmetic Dentist Super
Hero. He could ask her for advice on whitening his
teeth. We all were still puzzled by her comments, *"Modern Dentistry is Dead Wrong,"* and... *"Americans are
Drowning in a Sea of Toxic Teeth Bleach."*

Braen did just that, and during the next few months
he had weekly email exchanges with his new pal. He
discovered very interesting information about her and
what she does. She also was very interested in Braen's
and our whole family's incorporation of a purist natural
organic lifestyle. She had been gradually transforming
her personal life from the traditional standard American
diet of burger, fries, and coke. Fast food McDrive-ins
became taboo, and she had begun avoiding all restaurants, because she had no idea how the chef was
prepping her meal. She was now preparing most of her
food at home and was just as curious about our family's
lifestyle as we were interested in her knowledge about

21

teeth whitening. Organic food, herbs, and supplements were now replacing boxed, bagged, and canned "fake" food, which she now realized could only give her "fake" health.

Braen discovered that although his dentist buddy was becoming a purist at home, she had not been able to incorporate her new ideals into her Cosmetic Dental Practice. I understood the problem she was struggling with. When your source of income is creating a million dollars net income a year for you, there is a strong tendency not to disrupt the wheels that are moving the business. After all, her traditional dental practice purchased the beautiful, lush property in Ecuador. She would soon be retiring comfortably in the relative luxury of tropical rain forests, hidden waterfalls, organic fruit, and vegetables growing wild in her land, plus... enjoying the misty mountain peaks to hike for spiritual purification.

I don't believe at this time there are many dental business models practicing Holistic Dental Health Care while grossing 5 million dollars a year. It is understandable that our new dentist friend would more than hesitate to change the focus of her dental business from what she had developed over 25 years of hard work. She also was in the process of selling her practice to her new associate, and the timing could not have been worse to incorporate therapies such as homeopathic remedies, herbal immune boosters, muscle testing, and mercury vapor protective measures.

As I write this chapter, I would like to say that our dentist friend did not want her name to be publicly revealed. She had shared with us very personal and confidential information. Many of her statements about traditional dentistry were openly bold, confrontational, and most likely would jeopardize her standing within the dental community. State Dental Regulating Boards have been known to discipline and/or revoke dental licenses of dentists for making health related claims similar to hers. She was not going to jeopardize in any way or manner the sale of her 5 million dollar practice.

From here on, I will refer to our brave dentist friend as Dr. Q, and... the next few chapters will reveal her discoveries about teeth bleaching I personally found nearly unbelievable.

And **THEY WORK!**

I now understand why...

"MODERN DENTISTRY IS DEAD WRONG"

and why

"Americans are Drowning in Teeth bleach"

In this book you will discover...

**THE MOST POWERFUL AND
ONLY PRACTICAL ADVICE AVAILABLE
for A MORE NATURAL AND HOLISTIC
APPROACH TO TEETH WHITENING.**

Chapter 5

The Most Powerful and
Only Practical Advice Available

Dr. Q graduated tops in her class, Magna Cum Laude, and was the class valedictorian. She established one of the most successful Cosmetic Dentistry practices in the State of New York. Plus... she received numerous professional awards for her knowledge and skills in changing and perfecting smiles. Actors, models, celebrities, and business moguls came to her for Smile Makeovers.

Dr. Q's business success, however, was just one very visible aspect of her life, and she was a master at it. Secretly, behind closed doors, she was investigating a

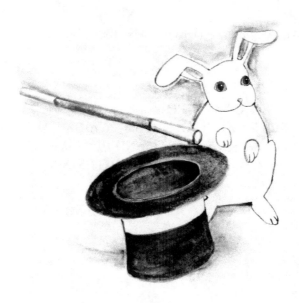

different lifestyle. Smile Makeovers became an illusion she could create as would a magician in star studded Las Vegas. Her heart began to quiver when she realized her life's work was mostly a "cover-up" of insecure psyches. Over time the thrill of magic and the applause of the audience began to wear off. Dr. Q wanted to be more than a 'magician'.

Dr. Q wondered where the word "health" fit into her uniquely successful practice of dentistry. After all, she originally became a dentist in order to help improve people's dental health. Somewhere in time the word "health" bent and twisted into the word "wealth", and her practice began to focus more on "Wealth".

The wheel of life does keep turning, and several years ago Dr. Q began to search into herself for the meaning of health. After spending at least 20,000 hours in research and over $250,000 of her hard earned money she finally made the determination that Modern Dentistry is Dead Wrong.

Dr. Q also wondered if there was a deep seated psychological reason behind her patients' desire to change their smiles. They would come into her office with teeth as white as Santa's beard and claim they looked yellow. They seemingly were obsessed with the pursuit of a whiter than white, maximum dazzle smile. In fact, according to the American Academy of Cosmetic Dentistry, teeth whitening is the No. 1 requested cosmetic dental procedure.

"People seem to be a little out of control. In fact, our whole society seems to be out of control when you analyze the quality of life people in America are living."

Dr. Q recognized this disorder in her own life, and she began to correct it with great success. However, she was so close to retiring and depending on the sale of her dental practice for retirement income that she could not find the courage to bring "health" back into her Magic Show at this time.

After nearly a quarter million dollars invested in 20,000 hours of continuing education, Dr. Q realized she had unearthed some very valuable, hidden, and controversial information about her specialty of cosmetic dentistry. She desperately wanted to unleash these awesome revelations to the world, but she did not have the time to organize her notes into readable form.

One night as she was flipping through her notes, Dr. Q prayed for direction and a thought popped into her mind. It was outlandish, but… the following day Braen received an email asking if he would be interested in transferring her notes into a readable book form. She would give him a salary, and he could create this book in his spare time.

At age 17, Braen was close to being his own man, but this request floored him. The income was tempting; however… he was a little insecure with his ability to complete the task. He asked for my advice.

I told him, *"This is your Best Day Ever! Go for it, and shout YES! If you have any questions, or need help with this amazing adventure, I'll be more than happy to help."*

In my mind I was thinking about how busy my life already was. In my heart I felt a serious debt to Dr. Q for saving my son. I would do anything for Dr. Q, and helping Braen write Dr. Q's book was the smallest gesture to show my deep appreciation.

Braen accepted the challenge, he was victorious, and… when it was over, he was a changed human being for the better. I helped him whenever he needed advice, and at the end I felt at peace.

The remaining chapters of this book reveal a distillation of the notes of Dr. Q. They may seem outlandish, but here's the best kept secret of all...

I WAS SHOCKED!!!

but everything in her notes works! They are packed with useful advice. I hope you enjoy, and benefit from, Dr. Q's unmatched wisdom when you read about...

A MORE NATURAL AND HOLISTIC
APPROACH TO TEETH WHITENING.

Chapter 6

A More Natural and
Holistic Approach to Teeth Whitening

In the following chapters I will reveal some of
Dr. Q's and my favorite teeth whitening secrets. These
are pearls that even some dentists don't know. You
will discover hidden revelations that your dentist may
NEVER tell you about whitening teeth. Braen, Jake,
myself, and my entire extended family and friends,
contributed our own independent research. We tried
everything that you will read in this book. Together with
Dr. Q's professional experience and advice the Brighte-
Smythe family has created what I believe is the BEST
SOURCE of teeth whitening information anywhere in
the world.

I have learned from Dr. Q a BETTER option than
professional office bleaching—and it COSTS LESS than
store bought bleaching products. You will be amazed
and shocked with this breakthrough formula that delivers MAXIMUM WHITENING in a MORE NATURAL,
HOLISTIC, and SAFE way… for just pennies a day.

You'll learn my ULTIMATE TEETH BLEACHING
TREATMENT. It's a solution so simple and effective it's
positively revolutionary…

I'll reveal to you what I do to prevent tooth decay,
gum disease, and how I whiten my own teeth. I will also
address safety issues, toxic side effects, and how teeth
whitening when done correctly may actually improve
your health.

A More Natural and Holistic Approach to Teeth Whitening

I want you to know that what I consider the world's best and safest teeth bleaching method isn't expensive. In fact, I could call it a 10 CENT CURE for our multi-million-dollar teeth whitening industry.

My Favorite Do-It-Yourself Teeth Whitening Cure

That's what my research suggests—a Teeth Whitening Cure for tooth decay, gum disease, and stained teeth. But that's not all! My system could very well be a miracle cure for...

- Gum abscess.
- Fever Blisters.
- Mouth ulcers.
- Oral herpes.
- Wisdom tooth pain.
- TMJ pain.
- Teeth on the verge of needing a root canal.

...and more!

It may be a powerful weapon against...

- Heart Disease
- Diabetes
- Arteriosclerosis
- Fibrous scar tissue
- Joint Pain
- Cancer

...and more revealed in the next few chapters!

So... what IS this awesome new powerhouse? Is it some ultra-risky drug that stills needs years of testing and tinkering? Is this a teeth bleaching method I have to pay hundreds of dollars for?

Not at all! In fact, what I have discovered is a more natural, holistic way to whiten my teeth, PLUS... improve my over all health, including teeth, gums, bone, and all the major organs of my body.

What I discovered is that teeth whitening isn't just a cosmetic procedure. It is a KEY life enhancing healing miracle.

That's right!
**The healing miracle of
Teeth Bleaching...**

I came to this realization when I noticed...

Glug!
Americans are drowning in a
toxic sea of bleaching gel!

Millions of Americans have had in-office dentist supervised bleaching.

50–100 million teeth bleaching kits have been sold throughout the world since 2001. This includes from pharmacies, at general retail stores, and on the Internet.

The following statistics are presented by manufacturers such as Colgate-Palmolive and Procter and Gamble.

There have been a reported adverse incident rate of 0.005% (1 report for every 20,000 kits sold). The vast majority of adverse events reported were oral soft tissue irritation and tooth sensitivity, which are transient and generally mild. American dentists have found that 2 out of 3 bleaching patients report mild and transient tooth sensitivity. Some people experience intolerable sensitivity and must stop the treatment. Unpublished comments have been, "I got a horrible toothache" and... "my dentist burned the **** out of my gums. My research shows that many people do not 'admit' intolerable sensitivity. The numbers are 'in fact' higher. Two of my best friends reported extreme teeth sensitivity episodes after professional bleaching applications. They didn't tell their dentists; they just never went back. There are many unreported negative side effects to teeth bleaching. Some of my children's classmates also had bad experiences. The experiences of my two closest friends are one reason I wanted to find a better and safer way to bleach teeth.

Hello? Does 2 out of 3 "mild, intolerable, transient, horrible, burned the **** tooth sensitivity" seem 'safe' to you? These are patients supervised by dentists in their dental offices. I also would question reports from big corporate giants that sell millions and millions of dollars of teeth whitening and bleaching products. Their "honest objective" studies reporting 'few' adverse reports might be twisted to increase sales dollars. After all, some dentists say they were involved in the toxic fluoride cover-up conspiracy.

Oh, I'm sorry. You didn't know that fluoride in our toothpaste and drinking water may be toxic to various organs of the body? End point studies with fluoride show cancer in every single animal tested. I have information on poison fluoride in the following chapters. You might want to keep reading to get this information. I'll also reveal the way I safely bleach and whiten my teeth without harsh, cruel, pain and sensitivity.

What's hurting YOU?

In 2007 the Council of European Dentists resolved that teeth whitening products containing 6% hydrogen peroxide (H_2O_2) are not safe to be sold over the counter but are safe to be used after the approval and under the supervision of a dentist. Teeth whitening products containing more that 6% H_2O_2 were not considered safe for use by the consumer.

This resolution is in stark contrast to what is happening in America. Over the counter retail products routinely contain more than 6% H_2O_2. Over the Internet one can buy teeth whitening products containing up to 15% H_2O_2.

In my opinion, these products may be hazardous to your health. In general, they have various toxic ingredients and / or dangerous 'tag along' byproducts. Yet... the Federal Drug Administration, and the American Dental Association, both seem to be in disagreement with European Council of Dentists. Somehow... the FDA, and ADA seem pretty confident in the safety of these products.

So what's up? FOLLOW THE MONEY! Cosmetic dentistry today is THE biggest money maker for American dentists. Teeth whitening products are making a fortune for companies such as Crest and Colgate.

A More Natural and Holistic Approach to Teeth Whitening

Americans are in a wild craze whitening their teeth. We can't make them white 'enough'. I call it the American White-Teeth Dream!

On the contrary, Europeans seem more inclined to let Mother Nature take its course. They don't seem to be interested in artificially changing the way they look. The teeth whitening market in Europe has not taken off as it has in America. In other words, Americans seem 'a bit' more easily persuaded to imitate Hollywood, and... there is MONEY to be made here.

I'm not one to put a lid on free enterprise. I believe in it strongly. However, I want my research open to the public so that you have access to important, not well known, information you'll want to consider, in 'opposition' to a lot of the 'hype' you've been getting. This information will enable you to make better decisions about the health of your teeth, gums, bone, and in general your whole body. I want you to know what I have discovered about the dangers of teeth whitening products on the market, and... what I myself am doing to safely whiten my teeth. I want you to understand the theory behind my discovery of the healing miracle of teeth whitening.

Continue READING, and You'll Soon Discover these Secrets!

You'll have access to the enlightening information I've accumulated from Dr. Q's 20,000 hours of research. You'll have the answers the Brighte-Smythe family discovered to all the questionable safety issues listed above. And... you'll see in detail what I do to safely and effectively whiten my teeth.

Plus you'll learn...

- Why you need 2 different teeth cleaning substances...
  1 for days you bleach, and 1 for days you don't
  bleach.
- The most advanced toothbrush you can buy today,
  and why it is the safest to use when you bleach.
- An ancient Ayurvedic tradition for killing disease
  causing bugs that make their home in gum pockets.
- The best antioxidants to use for neutralizing the
  effects of free radicals created during bleaching.
- How to get maximum oxygen absorption into your
  teeth, gums, and oral soft tissues during bleaching.
- Why I use an ancient Tibetan herb to boost the blood
  circulation to the pulp and nerve of the teeth.
- Pathways of chi energy through the teeth that are
  purified during the bleach process.
- Can you really detox teeth?
- Why the color of your teeth is unique to you, and how
  they became the color they are.
- Cavities are not caused by sugar.
- How bleaching my way changes an unhealthy acid
  mouth into a healthier alkaline pH.
- Why your mitochondria play an important role during
  bleaching.
- Why brushing with most toothpastes does next to
  nothing to prevent cavities..., nor gum disease.
- What exactly causes teeth to look old and discolored.
- How Russian submarines are connected with whitening teeth.

- A novel and significant cosmetic toothpaste found in Europe but not available in the U.S. IT works great for those unexpected emergencies when you didn't have time to whiten your teeth.
- Is 'mom' the reason for the color of your teeth?
- How low metabolic oxygen, inflammation, toxicity, infections, nutritional and hormonal deficiencies, and decreased physical fitness affect the color and health of your teeth.

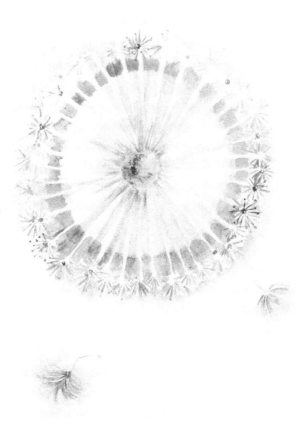

Stop Reading Here!

If you want "PIANO KEY" White Teeth, then… leave now and continue searching the Internet. I'm not going to scam you with a Magic Potion that will turn teeth white, whiter, whitest. I'm sharing with you my discovery for whitening teeth in a safe, healthy way. You'll see that the system I developed is holistic oriented with my health and the health of my teeth in mind. Many of today's modern whitening methods might pass the DUMBEST BLEACH TEST, but I believe my system is extra gentle, cheaper, safer, and healthier. I want my teeth to look naturally young, youthful, vibrant, elegantly whiter, and sparkling clean. You are going to see a sprightly zing in my smile, and it is going to carry me on my way to success in all aspects of my life.

I'm not into *refrigerator shocking white* and it's been nice knowing you… **Good Luck!** But, if you are open to new, innovative, and courageous thinking then read on about…

THE ONLY WAY I KNOW TO SURVIVE THE AMERICAN TEETH WHITENING FIASCO…

Chapter 7

The Only Way I Know
to Survive the American Teeth Whitening Fiasco

Teeth whitening is the leading dental procedure requested by people under the age of 20 and between the ages of 30 and 50. In the last 10 years alone, this procedure has exploded by 300 percent, according to The American Academy of Cosmetic Dentistry.

We live in a perfectionist culture where there is a mandate to be sexy. Dr. Q, as a dentist, believes that the pressure to have a sexy smile comes from our culture and to a large extent people around you including friends. The media is relentlessly focusing on celebrity sexy smiles making ordinary people feel inadequate when they can't achieve the same perfect dazzling whiteness of the Hollywood crowd. Everyday you see pictures and movies of Hollywood superstars with dazzlingly white teeth, and you wonder how you can live up to this standard. How can you be as glamorous as the runway Super Model?

When you have millions of people whitening their teeth, this sets new standards in our society for how "normal" teeth are supposed to look. Even if you have a healthy color, they may look yellow when compared to the flashy whites of movie stars and, now, the average person in America.

As further proof that culture drives our behavior the Kammu women in Laos and Vietnam painted their teeth black to be beautiful and cavity free. Nuts and wood were burned and the soot collected had a viscous quality. The fresh black soot was then applied to teeth with finger tips. Today, due to the influence of western culture on the eastern world, this practice has been discontinued with the younger generation. It is now known only among the elderly.

In my opinion the promotion and desire to live up to Hollywood's expectations is deviant and pathological behavior. It is our consumerist society, with its multi-billion-dollar cosmetic dentistry and medical surgery industry, that is behind the trend playing on peoples' insecurities.

Please don't misunderstand me. It IS good to feel attractive and sexy. I am all for it, support it, and will do everything I can to help the world become a billion times more attractive and sexy. But... when you have your teeth whitened, is there a sexy feeling deep within your heart pouring love and glamor outward through your smile? Or... is it only a superficial change happening? Are you really drawing into your heart the feeling of lack of attractiveness from the artificial changes in your teeth? Are you missing love in your life, and trying to attract it from others by deception? Wouldn't it be better to have all those wonderful, warm, huggy-snuggy feelings already within yourself, and then... give love freely to the world?

This is what I have discovered. To be authentic and sexy is our natural birthright. Every baby born, if born healthy, has the most attractive loving smile God could ever create. As the baby grows into adulthood, if he or she remains healthy, the individual's teeth will continue to shine forth and mature into a sexy, bright, dashing, glamorous smile.

The problem arises when that cute little baby matures into a young adult and then an adult. So often he/she loses health and subsequently a beautiful smile. I believe it is not possible to have a natural God given attractive smile unless a person is healthy in all ways. The best way to become attractive and sexy is first to regain your health. As you become healthier, the attractive and sexy will follow. This is what my research has uncovered.

Unfortunately, the Hollywood organism betrays us in every way. We believe that we must become just like the puppets on their stage. When we ignore our health and well-being we also lose our sparkling healthy smile. Rather than regain it through good healthy lifestyle changes, we have been convinced that a Hollywood Smile Make Over is the best way. It is fast, furious, and outwardly beautiful, but... it does the soul very little good.

The Magic Show Ends Here, Let Beauty Shine Through

The public is not usually aware that every picture of a superstar displayed in magazines, newspapers, books, and Internet is doctored with artistic air brushing to paint on the perfect bright smile. Digital technology makes this even easier, so that no matter what minor defect shows up in the photo it can be artificially changed to look perfect. Most celebrities do not have perfect smiles. They just look glamorous in print and electronic media after the magic make up is applied. Their personal artists touché up the photos. This is truly a magic show with deception at every corner, and the dentist plays a major role in the performance.

This quote from Dr. Q says it all:

"Many celebrities years ago had their teeth professionally bleached. Now with the advent of superbly thin veneers there are a huge number of superstars that display a perfect white smile because they asked their dentist to veneer their teeth. I know, because after 25 years of practicing cosmetic dentistry, I have become an expert at bleaching and veneering teeth for these very same unique, popular, and powerful people."

"I will admit that being a famous dentist artist is deeply satisfying and financially lucrative. I believe, though, that I have evolved beyond physical artistry, and I now have enough money. I am becoming more concerned with inner artistry. This is where true health and well being blossoms from deep within the body. As you restore health, your teeth will also return to their original angelic nature."

The following chapters will reveal to you my discoveries of how teeth are involved in regenerating health. I believe I have a formula to whiten teeth safely, naturally, and holistically. In the process... the teeth will detoxify unnatural, toxic chemicals, and substances. I will also explain exactly what it means to detox teeth and how the process is connected with improved health. I am convinced that if you detox your teeth, your overall health will improve. The body is a whole living breathing organism, and the teeth are intimately involved in the biology of being.

I will show you how I do this for myself. I practice what I preach. I detox my teeth regularly and as a result they have a brilliant natural shine while my overall health continues to regenerate. My entire family whitens their teeth with this detox formula. When you walk into my home there is a glowing halo of love smiling at every turn.

It does work!

However, before I reveal my formula I would like to share with you...

INCREDIBLE SHOCKING TOOTH TRUTHS

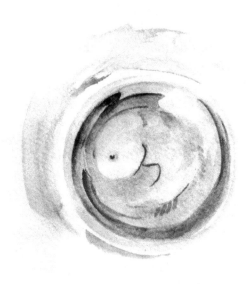

Chapter 8

Incredible Shocking Tooth Truths

It's important to me to share with you my teeth whitening formula, but first I would like to talk with you about veneers. The following story was related to me by Dr. Q.

"This all started over 20 years ago when a drop dead gorgeous blue eyed blond told me she wanted Hollywood veneers to whiten her teeth. This beautiful and charming 24 year old was a financial investment broker and she felt whiter teeth would help advance her career.

When I examined her teeth, I saw that she had perfect dentition, beautiful arch form, balanced occlusion, with no fillings and no tooth decay. In other words, she had teeth that I would give my right arm for.

But what about her tooth color? Beautiful and youthful Vita Shade A1. Shade A1 is usually seen in the healthy harmonious natural color of a young 12 year old. A1 is not 'white' but it is the perfect shade that many dentists try to duplicate for a youthful smile.

This young lady wasn't satisfied, because she had seen pictures of Hollywood Stars with 'white' teeth. She also knew that these stars had cosmetic veneers to cover their teeth and she wanted to belong to that small group of successful models and actors. Bleaching was just so "been there, done that."

I was stunned by her request. I tried to convince her that although she would be happy with the white color, cosmetic veneers would permanently deform her teeth. I told her that today she is a free and healthy person but if she finds a dentist to place veneers she would forever be a slave to that dentist, and... the veneers could potentially harm her health.

People are not aware that most veneers require grinding and permanent deformation of the enamel. They discolor with time, may chip and break, require regular maintenance, and will have to be replaced in the future. This will cost a considerable amount of money as one ages. In a manner of speaking, a person that has veneers placed will become a 'cash cow' for the dentist.

Speaking with this young lady, who was shrewd with finance and investments, I thought that if I focused on the long term cost, she might reconsider. What, I asked her, would she do if in the future she lost her job, a veneer broke, and she did not have the money to repair it?

Her response: 'Sure, as if I'm going to be a bag lady someday'!"

STEP INTO THE FABULOUS FUTURE OF COSMETIC VENEERS!

"15 years after my meeting with the young lady a 48 year old man walks into my office. He asks me to extract all his teeth and make him dentures. I examine his mouth and see about a dozen discolored, chipped, broken, and unsightly veneers. The teeth are vital and fairly healthy, however, the veneers look like Shrek lost in a Halloween Nightmare.

This gentleman is a former CEO of his self made software company. He has 6 kids, 4 of them in orthodontic braces. His company went belly up. He has no job. His once handsome smile of perfect veneers has turned into a horrible mask of dread. They all need to be replaced.

The problem is that this man is a floss thread away from bankruptcy. He has no money to repair his veneers. He feels that pulling all his teeth and getting fitted for dentures is his only alternative. I admire him, though, for putting his family's welfare above his own. Would you pull all your teeth, and gum it for the rest of your life, in order to keep your kids in braces?

So there you have an example of the potential risk you take when you try to imitate Hollywood "White Smile" Stars, and veneer your teeth."

Incredibly Shocking Tooth Truths!

More importantly to me is that the health of the teeth is compromised with veneers. Veneered teeth may shorten the life expectancy of both the teeth, and… the person wearing them.

Did you know that teeth are a living breathing part of the human anatomy? You may have heard that George Washington had wooden teeth but believe me, your teeth are not dead wood stumps planted into jaw bone. Teeth are very much alive!

Hey JAKE! When's the mulch coming?

Yes, and just like a giant oak tree, teeth:
- Grow from a seed and develop within an embryo in the mother's womb.
- Are affected by the mother's emotions, chemistry, nutrition, and love.
- Pop up from the gums at a pretty predictable time during infancy.
- Have roots that draw vital life giving nutrients from the blood stream.
- Have a circulatory system within the roots, trunk, and branches that we can call periodontal space, root, and crown.
- Breath oxygen similar to an oak tree breathing carbon dioxide.
- Like tree bark, teeth have a protective outer covering called cementum and enamel. This covering can be scratched and damaged during regular teeth cleanings, tooth brushing, and day to day food, drink, and chemicals.
- Teeth flex and move during chewing as does the giant oak when the wind chews it in a storm.
- Teeth sweat through a mineral exchange with saliva as do the leaves of an oak tree when they exchange minerals with the dew and environment.
- Teeth can also withstand the tremendous impact of biting and accidental blows to the jaw. Have you ever seen an oak tree wrestle with a tornado or hurricane? Thunder vibrating it to its roots, wind biting its trunk toward the ground, lightning electrifying ever cell in its body, and even capturing a mobile home in its branches?
- Teeth feel, bleed, hear, smell, taste, snap, crackle, pop.

Teeth are alive

If you crazy glue the face of your tooth with a plastic or porcelain veneer-like-shingle, do you think it 'might' affect the way that tooth breathes and drinks? Do you think it might breathe 'less' oxygen and drink 'fewer' minerals from the saliva? I would especially caution athletes against cosmetic veneers. You need every molecule of Oxygen and Mineral to maximize performance.

Think of it like this. When you shingle the roof of your home, does this keep wind, rain, and snow from penetrating the roof? And how long before you need to rip out old worn and torn shingles to make your roof look new again... 15–20 years? Well, that's probably a little longer than the lifetime of a veneer. Yes, your roof shingle will probably have a longer lifetime than your cosmetic veneer!

Your tooth is not a house made of dead wood, steel, aluminum, and plastic. Your tooth is alive and connected to your body. It needs all its functions working perfectly, if you want it to last your entire life. Teeth are living organisms and need to "sweat" in order to expel their metabolic wastes. A tooth whose entire surface is blocked with varnish, veneers, and crowns cannot expel and detox its wastes, leading to more toxic waste over time. When you place cosmetic veneers on your teeth, you are burdening them with an impervious wall of glue, plastic, and porcelain. I would guess that 25% of their life force has been affected. There are no long term studies of 50 years or more examining safety and how this affects your life and the life of your teeth. Believe me, according to recent medical and scientific research, you are most likely going to live MUCH longer… maybe even another 75–100 years.

So here's what I want you to try. Go to your neighborhood Gnome Depot and buy a gallon can of wood deck sealer. Spray this sealer to cover 25% of the crown of your neighbor's tree. Make sure it's greener than nature intended. We are trying to improve on nature, right? We want the greenest green money can buy— high density green with THX.

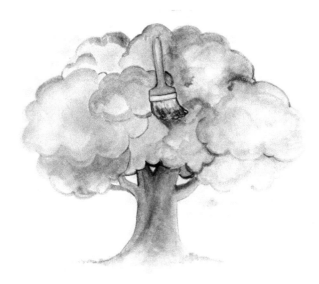

In about a week tell me what you see. Is your neighbor still speaking with you?

I admit veneers on teeth won't produce such an immediate response. It will be more subtle. I am convinced it puts a physical and chemical burden on the body that will play a role in disease later in life. I want you to know that there is a high probability that you will live to at least 120 years. There are also scientific theories that predict today we have people among us that will live at least 1000 years. Do everything you can to keep your teeth your whole life, and stay as healthy as possible

I, myself, am avoiding veneers at all cost. I'll show you what I do to prevent myself from wanting or ever needing veneers. Bleaching teeth is far more natural, safer, and healthier when done in a way that blends proven ancient health secrets with 21st century science. Plus there are many health benefits to teeth bleaching, which I will soon explain.

In the next chapter you'll learn a part of my teeth detox formula, and why it is a must to have...

THE BEST DEFENSE AGAINST DANGEROUS BLEACH PRODUCTS

Chapter 9

The Best Defense Against Dangerous Bleach Products

Hydrogen peroxide is the active ingredient in almost all bleaching products. Other substitutes include urea peroxide, carbamide peroxide, calcium peroxide, magnesium peroxide, sodium perborate, sodium percarbonate, sodium hydroxide, potassium hydroxide, calcium hydroxide, and triethanol amine, and EDTA.

Wow! This is a long list of bleaching chemicals. Are they safe under all conditions in the mouth?

If you have been reading recent news articles about the dangers of hydrogen peroxide, you might be wondering what makes hydrogen peroxide so dangerous? Actually, this is a topic of great controversy. In general the scientific community agrees that at certain concentrations, in different environments, and within various biochemical processes, hydrogen peroxide $\{H_2O_2\}$ can cause aging, disease development, or death.

The reason H_2O_2 is harmful is that when it reacts with different substances it creates water $\{H_2O\}$ and a highly reactive oxygen $\{O_2\}$ (or a superoxide anion $\{O_2^{\cdot-}\}$, a peroxide $\{O_2^{-2}\}$, a hydroxyl radical $\{\cdot OH\}$, or a hydroxyl ion $\{OH^-\}$) called a "free radical." This reactive oxygen or "free radical" is a strong oxidizer, not very stable, and creates chain reactions of more free radicals. I will later explain in more detail about how H_2O_2 works, what oxidizers do, and their good and bad effects in the body. Suffice it now to say that the reason we hear so much about antioxidants in the news media is that antioxidants are defense mechanisms to protect the body from free radical oxidizers and the damage they inflict. The body has to have sufficient antioxidants to do battle with free radicals in order to prevent aging, disease, or death. So understand that there are some safety concerns about too many oxidants and not enough antioxidants. Free radicals can cause aging, disease, and even death. The very young, immune compromised, and elderly are more sensitive to the damaging free radical effects of hydrogen peroxide.

You should also know that all teeth whitening bleach gels have one or more of either hydrogen peroxide, urea peroxide, carbamide peroxide, magnesium peroxide, and calcium peroxide. These peroxides create free radicals that can be either harmful or beneficial to you. The free radicals oxidize interprismatic extrinsic staining within the tooth enamel. A correct understanding of their properties is important if you plan to whiten your teeth.

Protect yourself from possible harmful effects of bleaching gels.

My solution is so simple and effective it's positively revolutionary...

As you now know, hydrogen peroxide can be hazardous to your health; however, it is a basic necessity of life. It is found everywhere on earth in very low concentrations including the atmosphere surrounding the earth and in waters, rain, and snow. The sun's energy ionizes H_2O_2 found in the atmosphere creating free radicals called hydroxyl radicals (OH). Tiny even by molecular standards, the hydroxyl radical (OH) is so small that 10 billion billions would fit in a raindrop. It is continuously replenished during the day. These molecules have been described as "the single most important cleansing agent in the earth's atmosphere." They are necessary for natural air cleansing and toxin removal.

Hydroxyl radicals are the atmosphere's natural cleansing filter. They are found naturally in abundance in outdoor fresh air, with high concentrations found in forested mountain areas. The hydroxyl radical acts as an oxidizing agent. It removes several greenhouse gases and other pollutants from the atmosphere. Hydroxyls purge more than half the sulfur dioxide added to the air by smokestacks, volcanoes and other sources. Hydroxyls are why our planet hasn't choked itself to death and the reason we can live in our cities.

Scientists have developed a unique air purifier which, according to independent research, can kill the viruses H_1N_1 Swine Flu and H_5N_1 Bird Flu within minutes in any room or other enclosed space. It is also effective against the MRSA 'superbug' and other airborne bacteria and viruses:

The unit creates a continual supply of hydroxyl radicals, to destroy microbes including flu and cold viruses and bacteria, both in the air and on surface contact. When someone sneezes, the particles of mucus ejected are full of viruses. The hydroxyl radicals from the unit condense onto these particles and rapidly destroy the viruses. This same condensation effect takes place on contaminated surfaces, killing surface viruses and bacteria within a number of hours. The radical purifier destroys micro-organisms in the air by cutting holes in their cell walls.

Hydrogen peroxide is also a very important factor in your body's trillions of biochemical processes. In the human body, hydrogen peroxide is produced primarily in three places—the lung, gut, and thyroid gland.

Did you know that your own white blood cells produce hydrogen peroxide? Yes they do, and... lots of it. That is how they kill invading germs. It's your body's first and best defense against infectious bacteria, yeast, parasites, and viruses. The intense bubbling you see when you pour H_2O_2 on a cut or wound is the oxygen being released to destroy bacteria. Yes, H_2O_2 oxidizes these bad guys and bam! terminated. Even certain tumors are treated with hydrogen peroxide.

PLUS

Vitamin C helps fight infections by producing H_2O_2.

Gut Bacteria produce H_2O_2 to destroy harmful bacteria and viruses preventing colon disease, bladder infections, and a host of other ailments. Most strains of harmful bacteria cannot survive in the presence of oxygen or H_2O_2.

Enzyme Systems throughout the body are stimulated by H_2O_2. This increases metabolic rate, causes arterioles to dilate and increase blood flow to oxygen starved areas of the body.

Tissue Oxygen Levels are positively affected by H_2O_2.

Oxygen Starvation may be remedied with H_2O_2. We are living in an oxygen starved world, and our cells are screaming for more of it. Airborne toxins, chlorinated water, over-processed foods, cooking, rampant antibiotic use, synthetic fats, and hydrogenated byproducts all react with hydrogen peroxide limiting the amount that our tissues have to thrive on.

Zebra Fish demonstrate "natural bleach" which scientists believe may be a key to healing. When the tail fins of these fish were injured, a burst of hydrogen peroxide was released from the wound and into the surrounding tissue. Teams of white blood cells appear to respond to this chemical signal, arriving at the site of the wound to begin the healing process. H_2O_2 may signal human cells to heal in a similar way.

So it is commonly agreed that hydrogen peroxide within the individual body cells is essential for life. And when applied topically, everyone agrees on its effectiveness to treat infections. The controversy deals with ingesting the substance orally. I'll show you how I settled this dispute to my satisfaction.

If you hear your dentist say that teeth bleaching gels are perfectly safe and millions of people across America have bleached their teeth safely, he may be correct to a point. But when I look a little more closely I see a few issues about the "safely" part, and this is why I have developed what I believe to be a friendlier and safer solution. I'll demonstrate how I take advantage of the good properties of H_2O_2 to oxygenate and improve my health while at the same time whiten my teeth. I'll also tell you what I do to protect myself from the dangerous free radicals created by H_2O_2.

How Teeth Whitening May Save Your Life with...
The healing miracle of hydrogen peroxide

But Wait...
let's examine the sea of toxic bleach ingredients we are drowning in...

In 2007 the Council of European Dentists supported the opinion of the European Scientific Council on Consumer Products. Teeth whitening products containing between 0.1 and 6% hydrogen peroxide were not considered safe to be sold over the counter, but were safe if approved under the supervision of a dentist. Teeth whitening products over 6% were not considered safe for use by the consumer at any time.

In the United States, over the Internet, one can buy 35% carbamide peroxide which is equivalent to about 15% hydrogen peroxide. One has to ask why can we in America buy products over the Internet that have 15% hydrogen peroxide, while in Europe it is considered unsafe. I know of at least one country, England, that makes it illegal to sell these concentrations over the counter. I'll give you some answers in this book and show you how I safely use hydrogen peroxide to whiten my teeth and prevent disease pathogens from invading my body.

In an August 2004 meeting of head and neck surgeons, researchers reported on two patients, in their twenties, who developed advanced tongue cancer decades earlier than usual. The two patients had a history of repeated use of teeth whitening products. The researchers suspect that hydrogen peroxide in the whitening gels may be the culprit. Two people, however, is a ridiculously small study and more investigations are needed.

Conditions such as pre-existing tissue injury or the concurrent use of alcohol and/or tobacco while using teeth whiteners may also exacerbate their toxic effects. Hydrogen peroxide, even at concentrations as low as 3%, may be especially harmful to oral tissues if they have been previously injured.

All bleaching materials diffuse hydrogen peroxide through dentin. Long term treatment can present problems to the pulp. The dental pulp is vulnerable through exposed dentin in patients with receding gums, attrition, cervical abrasion, and leaking fillings. The gingiva may be exposed directly to hydrogen peroxide gels during treatment. This is all a bit technical, but the bottom line is that some investigators are very concerned about the safety of hydrogen peroxide in bleach gels. I feel pretty confident using H_2O_2 in my formula and I'll tell you why later.

Laboratory studies documented mercury release from mercury silver fillings when exposed to carbamide peroxide solutions. I am concerned about the toxic effects of mercury in silver fillings and solved this issue about 20 years ago. I replaced all my mercury silver fillings with white tooth colored bonded composite fillings.

Yes, I do have a mouth full of fillings. When I was younger I did not know how to prevent tooth decay, and I will guarantee to you that brushing with a fluoride toothpaste is not the answer. I had been using fluoride toothpaste the first 32 years of my life. My children have been using fluoride toothpaste until several years ago. We all have had cavities.

Jake and Braen are the only ones that have never had a cavity. I'm jealous, but there are several reasons why. I'll explain how my teeth whitening method helps stop tooth decay. I don't believe I'll ever get another cavity as long as I live a healthy life and follow ridiculously simple rules.

UV light-enhanced teeth bleaching, according to recent investigations, is not only a flimflam but is dangerous to your eyes and skin. Researchers found that bleaching damaged teeth and created exposed grooves on the enamel surface that make the teeth more vulnerable to mechanical stress.

Polyomylpyrrolidone and polyvinylpyrrolidone are thickening agents used in some bleach gels. Glycerin and/or propylene glycol and/or polyethylene glycol are also carrier agents.

Polyvinyl acetate (PVA) is a chemical that is used to make thermoplastic bleach trays.

PVA always has a trace residue of vinyl acetate, which can "out gas" from the plastic and lead to environmental and human exposure. But don't worry, say government officials. Only a "trace" amount leaks out into your mouth. Isn't that 'comforting'?

Ethylene vinyl acetate is the chemical that makes up of the popular footwear Crocs. Wouldn't you say that it looks very similar to polyvinyl acetate, the chemical that makes up common bleach trays? Remember that vinyl acetate made the Canadian government's toxic list.

Some people might say that having a bleach tray in your mouth may not be much different than sucking a Croc.

The Canadian government has declared vinyl acetate to be a toxic substance and, you guessed it, the chemical is in a host of consumer items such as bleach trays. Synonyms for vinyl acetate which is used to make polyvinyl acetate bleach trays are acetic acid ethenyl ester, acetic acid ethylene ether, acetoxyethene, 1-acetoxyethylene, ethenyl ethanoate, ethenyl acetate, vinyl acetate monomer, acetic acid vinyl ester, vyac, and zeset T.

Vinyl Acetate MSDS
Stability

Stable. Highly flammable. Incompatible with acids, bases, oxidizing agents, peroxides, chloro-sulfonic acid, ethylene imine, hydrochloric acid, oleum, nitric acid, sulfuric acid, 2-aminoethanol, light. Susceptible to polymerization; commercial product may be stabilized by the addition of hydroquinone.

Toxicology

Possible carcinogen. May affect fertility. Risk of irreversible effects. Possible mutagen. Harmful if swallowed, inhaled or absorbed through the skin. Severe eye irritant. May cause skin burns if trapped in contact with skin.

Studies have shown that often less than 50 percent of the whitener gel is present in bleach trays one hour after application. The amount of leakage may be even higher in over-the-counter whitening products in which the trays are not custom fitted by a dentist. Therefore, during the whitening process, the oral mucosa is exposed to high concentrations of peroxide. This may have negative consequences, but an argument can be made that hydrogen peroxide is rapidly metabolized in the oral cavity by superoxide dimutase, catalase, salivary peroxidase, ascorbic acid and other antioxidants and therefore does not have a significant clinical affect on the mucosa.

In my opinion, that may be true for a healthy young adult. If you are over the age of 25 and/or your health is compromised, I'm not certain your body can produce the necessary enzymes and antioxidants to fully protect you from H_2O_2.

WARNING! Hydrogen peroxide available at drug stores is 3% solution. In such small concentrations, it is less stable and decomposes faster. It is usually stabilized with acetanilide, a substance which has toxic side effects in significant amounts.

Chemicals in ordinary tap water or store bought distilled water may cause a chemical reaction that prematurely strips the extra oxygen atom from the hydrogen peroxide atoms. Your hydrogen peroxide then loses much of its bleaching effectiveness. I'll tell you how I get pure and safe hydrogen peroxide and how to preserve its potency.

As you read onward you'll have access to all the information I've accumulated from Dr. Q's 20,000 hours of research. You'll have the answers I've discovered through my own research to settle the questionable safety issues listed above. You'll see in detail what I do to safely and effectively whiten my teeth.

Keep on reading to learn more about...

HYDROGEN PEROXIDE...
STRAW HATS TO SPACE ROCKETS

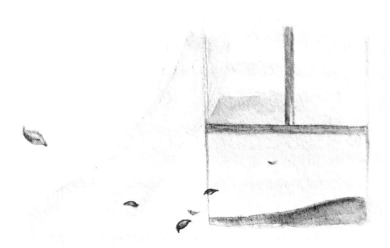

Chapter 10

Hydrogen Peroxide...
Straw Hats to Space Rockets

Hydrogen Peroxide (H_2O_2) was discovered in 1818 by Louis Jacque Thenard. Its oldest commercial use was for bleaching straw hats. Its most common use is to clear pollution from water and air. Other common uses are:

- Fight unfriendly bacterial colonies.
- Support bacterial growth to enhance contaminated soil and water.
- Bleach paper, cloth, teeth, hair.
- Disinfect scrapes, cuts, and gum disease.
- Propel Russian submarines.
- Jump start rockets and steer space satellites.

Hydrogen Peroxide is a clear colorless liquid that easily mixes with water. It is able to kill bacteria, fungi, viruses, parasites, and some types of tumor cells. Small amounts are found in rain and snow. It is an important part of plant life and is found in many vegetables and fruit. It has also been found in many of the healing springs of the world including Fatima in Portugal and Lourdes in France.

Hydrogen peroxide can irritate the eyes, skin and mucous membranes. Exposure of the eyes to concentrations of 5% or more can result in permanent eye damage. Skin exposure can cause painful blisters, burns, and skin whitening. Handle with care all concentrations of H_2O_2 greater than 3%.

Hydrogen peroxide readily crosses biological membranes. Because it reacts slowly with organic substances, it can travel considerable distances into biological systems. The greatest drawback of peroxide bleaching gels is the tendency of the chemical to decompose. Heavy metal ions—especially manganese, iron, and copper—catalyze the decomposition of H_2O_2. These ions greatly reduce the efficiency of the bleaching process. Thus chelating agents such as EDTA are used to form complexes with heavy metals and prevent their interference. This improves bleach ability to dissipate further into the tooth and reduces brightness reversion.

Hydrogen peroxide is identified with the words oxidation and reduction, The simplest way to define oxidation is "the loss of electrons from an atom, compound, or molecule." In general terms it means a chemical reaction of a substance with oxygen (O_2) or an oxygen-containing material which adds oxygen atoms(s) to the compound being oxidized.

$$H_2O_2 = H_2O + O_2$$

Oxidation reactions are usually exothermic. This means hydrogen peroxide can cause other materials including fire to burn more fiercely. When you bleach teeth, the hydrogen peroxide penetrates porous enamel and then "burns" and discolors the stained organic colloidal matrix.

Teeth bleaching almost always utilizes the power of liquid hydrogen peroxide (H_2O_2), Carbamide peroxide gel, however, is the most common way to carry the H_2O_2 into the teeth. Calcium peroxide is a solid peroxide found in teeth cleaning pastes and chewing gum. It is minimally effective in keeping teeth stain free.

Carbamide peroxide is white or yellowish in color. It is close to insoluble in water but will dissolve in acid to form hydrogen peroxide. When in contact with water it will immediately begin to decompose releasing oxygen. The oxygen is the active energy behind bleaching teeth. The teeth will turn whiter when a sufficient diffusion of oxygen passes through the enamel.

Now that we have talked a little about hydrogen peroxide and oxidation let's see what's so frightening about...

Oxidative Damage

Tick...Tick...Tick...BOOM!

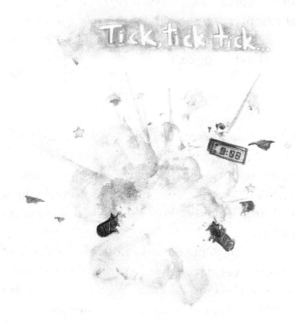

Chapter 11

Tick...Tick...Tick...BOOM!

What I'm about to tell you is incredibly important if you plan to bleach your teeth! Balance is the key to life. Your body spirals into and out of oodles and oodles of oxidant/antioxidant chemical reactions. I urge you to do everything possible to prevent upsets to the delicate oxidant/antioxidant balance within your body systems. Bleaching your teeth without this awareness may lead to a shorter life expectancy.

To clarify what I'm trying to say here, let's begin with the basic theory of oxidation. Please take a moment to read the following unusual story of what is happening in your body. Braen gets much of the credit for developing this chapter with his knowledge of martial arts and science fiction

IT'S WAR! Tiny bacteria, fungus, viruses, and chemicals have broken through your defensive line of immunity. These dangerous villains often take refuge deep inside your body where they remain hidden and dormant until they find an opportunity to invade other body parts. These infections can linger for months, years, or even a lifetime. They may never kill you, though infection can compromise your quality of life.

Conventional wisdom warns you to prepare for these invasions by "tuning" and revving your immune system up to full power. You may have read that nothing science has discovered can match the awesome inner healing powers of your immune system—when it is operating at full capacity.

What do you do when critters, bugs and chemicals not necessarily overpower your immune system, but use espionage, mind meld, psychic control, and other secretive spy mechanisms to work with, control, and then attack the healthy cells in your body?

I compare this horrible treachery with the traditional Eastern Martial Arts theory of using your opponent's energy to defeat him. Yes, your immune system might look as invincible as Bruce Lee, but a slick invader like Jackie Chan could carry a big bag of tricks that is capable of defeating the Master. With Drunken Kung Fu he can stick to you, infiltrate, and harness the almost unbelievable strength of your defending warriors. People flip when I suggest that hydrogen peroxide creates free radicals that can become Ninja like pathogens which have the ability to psychically power up your army to commit a coup mutiny with your own energy.

These tactics can be so overwhelming that...

Tick...Tick...Tick...BOOM!

...you become easily defeated, diseased, and die. Yes, there is a war being staged within you. Two of the major parties involved are oxidants and antioxidants. Whitening your teeth with hydrogen peroxide can be a tipping point in your favor. First you must be equipped with good knowledge and understanding of oxidation and antioxidants. Only then can you weigh the risk/benefit of oxidation with hydrogen peroxide. If you are not familiar with these concepts, then teeth whitening can be detrimental to your health. It can become the hidden Ninja that attacks your health... BOOM!...drops you to your knees.

Tick...Tick...Tick...BOOM!

As you now know... hydrogen peroxide, a strong oxidizer, can be hazardous to your health. It is, however, a basic necessity of life. Your immune system utilizes strong oxidizers such as H_2O_2 to inactivate pathogens. But H_2O_2 can also be a noxious oxidant. That's right! Hydrogen peroxide is VITAL to your health, as WELL as being a possible destructive agent to your life expectancy.

There is a constant, delicate interplay between oxidants and antioxidants occurring within you. Hydrogen peroxide, the active ingredient in teeth bleaching, is one of the major players on this stage. If you are on the path of radiant health and longevity, you should be aware of hydrogen peroxide and its role in oxidant/antioxidant reactions. You have to understand how to use the positive to eliminate the negative. You must play an active role in controlling hazardous H_2O_2 while supporting positive H_2O_2. It is critical that you understand how to use antioxidants to control noxious H_2O_2. This awareness must be present in all aspects of your life including teeth whitening.

This is where we set the stage for the Free Radical Theory of Aging...

FREE RADICAL... TERRORIST WITHIN!

65

The Teeth Whitening Cure

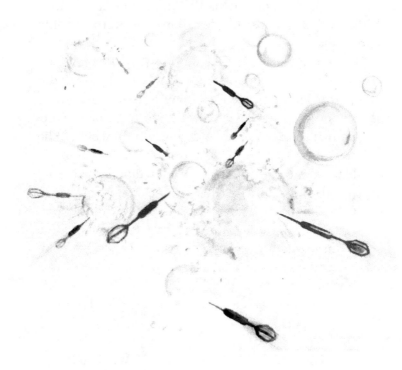

Chapter 12

Free Radical...Terrorist Within!

FACT... (negative effects)
- Hydrogen Peroxide is a strong oxidizer that creates Free Radicals.
- Free Radicals damage mitochondria cell membranes that may ultimately lead to Death.
- Bleaching Gels use hydrogen peroxide to Oxidize stains within teeth enamel ultimately creating Free Radicals.
- Free Radicals from Bleaching Gels cause Cell Death.

Therefore... Teeth whitening with bleach gels cause cell death and may be harmful to your health. – – – – – –

FACT... (positive effects)
+ Hydrogen Peroxide is a strong oxidizer that uses reactive oxygen to create Free Radicals.
+ Free Radicals and reactive oxygen Destroy and Eliminate Toxins from the teeth.
+ Bleaching Gels use hydrogen peroxide to Oxidize stains within teeth enamel ultimately Destroying and Eliminating Toxins from the teeth.

Therefore... Teeth whitening with bleach gels destroy and eliminate toxins from teeth and may be beneficial to your health. + + + + + +

+ As you can see, the free radicals that arise from teeth whitening bleach have both positive and negative consequences. They can cause cell death... vitally important to killing harmful bacteria, fungus, and virus. The reactive oxygen in bleach gel can also destroy and eliminate toxins that accumulate in the teeth enamel.

– However, bleach gels also create toxic free radicals, which may damage mitochondria cell membrane resulting in the death of cells essential to human life.

Confused? Is teeth whitening safe (+) or is the process a terrorist within (−)?

Both, actually!

The hydrogen peroxide used in teeth whitening has both positive and negative reactions. My way of whitening teeth supports the positive and reduces the negative. I have developed a method to whiten my teeth so that I take advantage of all the positive benefits while reducing the negative impact of dangerous free radicals. I will explain in detail exactly how I do this. For now let's learn more about free radicals, oxidants, and antioxidants.

Free radicals may be produced inside the body through normal metabolism. Inhaling oxygen produces free radicals. 2–3% of the oxygen consumed by our cells is converted into free radicals. Free radicals may also be a response to toxins that enter the body from the environment through pollution such as cigarette smoke, automobile exhaust, industrial chemicals, and yes... bleach gel ingredients. The body has a defense mechanism against free radicals referred to as antioxidants.

If the amount of antioxidants in the body is not enough to combat the free radicals, then the DNA can be altered possibly leading to aging and degenerative diseases. The general syndrome identified with an overwhelming barrage of free radical damage is called...

...oxidative stress.

Oxidative stress can kill you. It can be a slow process or accelerate death rapidly. But sooner or later oxidative stress will damage tissue and lead to accelerated aging and disease. Pollution, toxins, food, and even exercise produce oxidants. The resulting stress and expressed emotions of the body-mind connection cause a multitude of chemical reactions to take place. These can overwhelm the body's natural equilibrium in favor of oxidative damage.

Stress is unavoidable in today's world. We are in constant exposure to stress from environmental and metabolic oxidation. Bleaching gel is just one more cracker in the box that can lead to the rot and rust due to oxidative stress in our body. In order to maintain balance we have to make a conscious effort to support the positive, and reduce the negative, effects of living in the modern world. Soon you will read exactly how I approach this dilemma when I whiten my teeth.

The following is a list of things that create free radical stress... in case these concepts are new to you:
- *Over eating, sugar, and poor nutrition from fast food restaurants.*
- *Artificial ingredients/preservatives in boxed, canned, and bagged foods.*

- *Electronic equipment, lights, cell phones, computers.*
- *Household cleaning chemicals.*
- *Alcohol and pharmaceutical drugs.*
- *Sun burning, too much exercise, and not enough exercise.*
- *Infection, disease, and aging.*

All living beings produce oxidative biochemicals, and nature has designed the perfect way to clear these toxic substances. It does this by providing molecules called antioxidants. Antioxidants quench free radicals, and every cell in the body has this superb ability to neutralize toxicity. Nature also provides antioxidants in the food, water, and air that surround us. Our environment is a miraculous source of antioxidants.

Hydrogen peroxide in bleaching gel contributes to free radical oxidative stress, and this is a major concern of mine. That is why I am spending a lot of time talking about antioxidants.

Let's keep in mind the following positives of H_2O_2:

- The body has enzymes that limit the amount of hydrogen peroxide by speeding up the break-down of hydrogen peroxide into water and oxygen. In humans these enzymes are present in nearly all cells. For instance, enzymes in the saliva process hydrogen peroxide very efficiently and are the primary defenses against peroxide produced by bacteria in the mouth.
- Mother's milk has a considerable amount of H_2O_2, which enhances the immature immunologic system of the newborn against infective foreign agents.
- Green tea, black tea, and especially instant coffee contain naturally occurring H_2O_2.

A number of clinics in the United States and Mexico use hydrogen peroxide therapy usually given by intravenous injection to treat illness, disease, and cancer on a routine basis. As you can see, the body uses H_2O_2 as a weapon against infections and disease. We can also supplement our body with antioxidants from the environment around us including food, drink, and air. The body also uses naturally occurring enzymes and antioxidants to cope with the dangers of hydrogen peroxide

Supplementing with antioxidants is a critical step I use when whitening my teeth. First of all, modern living almost guarantees that our body's natural source of antioxidants cannot neutralize all the free radicals in and around us. Plus... with age our body slowly loses its ability to manufacture sufficient antioxidants. Since each person is an individual, no one knows exactly at which age this becomes an issue. Most scientific theories, however, place age 25 as the turning point for the average person.

The body produces the enzyme catalase, which breaks down hydrogen peroxide into water and oxygen. Or at least it does for a while. As we age, catalase production tails off, leaving nothing to transform the hydrogen peroxide into chemicals the body can release.

Individuals with certain inherited genetic disorders, such as acatalasemia and G6PD deficiency are more vulnerable to the damaging effects of hydrogen peroxide than those without these disorders. This condition is characterized by small, painful ulcers in the gingival crevices and tonsillar lacunae, attributed to excess levels of hydrogen peroxide generated by various microorganisms in the mouth without normal destruction by the catalase enzyme.

71

The Teeth Whitening Cure

Xerostomia, or dry mouth, is a genetic disorder in which the salivary glands are less active than normal. Xerostomia is also a side effect of many pharmaceutical drugs and chemotherapy agents. A dry mouth would have insufficient catalase enzyme, which may affect the efficient break down of hydrogen peroxide in the mouth.

White blood cells kill parasites, bacteria, viruses, and fungi by using H_2O_2; however, prolonged infections can result in increased exposure of the body cells to H_2O_2, which may be harmful.

The world seems to have been caught up in the idea all biological oxidation is harmful because free-radicals may be produced. Free-radicals can cause lipid per-oxidation and membrane damage. Consequently many products containing antioxidants are being promoted to prevent peroxidation.

However, some researchers feel peroxidation serves a useful purpose in the biochemical balance and may need stimulating at times, instead of preventing. Researchers have suggested that small exposure to oxidative conditions may actually offer protection from acute doses. Studies actually suggest that we humans may be able to prolong the aging process by regularly exposing our bodies to minimal amounts of oxidants.

The technical word for this is adaption. It is an effect where a toxic substance acts like a stimulant in small doses but is an inhibitor in large doses. So it is probably true that small exposure to hydrogen peroxide may actually prolong your life by stimulating the adaption effect. The question remains as to how much exposure is too much?

The body has the ideal antioxidant defense system, but it becomes less effective as we age. As we age, the best protection against free radical damage is to supplement with nutrients like vitamins A, C, E, minerals like selenium, cofactors like Coenzyme Q10, carotenoids, flavonoids, N-acetyl cysteine (NAC), and herbs. These are some of the nutrients that I take to support me, especially when I bleach my teeth.

You can now see clearly that... at times hydrogen peroxide production within the body needs to be stimulated. And... at 'other' times the H_2O_2 "terrorist" needs to be "destroyed and taken out" in order to protect ourselves from its negative forces.

The following three statements should finally clarify why I am so concerned about teeth whitening with hydrogen peroxide:

1. *The International Agency for Research on Cancer has evaluated the carcinogenic potential of hydrogen peroxide and concluded that the data was considered insufficient for making a decision with regards to humans.*
2. *While hydrogen peroxide is not a 'proven' carcinogen, it does cause local inflammation and tissue irritation at high concentrations.*
3. *The complex interactions of the inflammatory response, combined with other factors, may have an unpredictable effect on tissues.*

Hydrogen peroxide does generate reactive hydroxyl radicals, which can produce oxidative DNA damage; but in humans these radicals are scavenged by the body's peroxidase mechanism and cellular stores of glutathione

and protein. However, this mechanism may be substan-
tially impeded, unless a person:

- is born into a healthy loving family that is living in
  the mountains or valley isolated from the physical
  and mental stresses of the 21st century.
- eats organic whole foods.
- drinks naturally pure uncontaminated spring water.
- breathes unpolluted air.
- sleeps in an environment free of electro-smog
  including cell phones, radios, televisions, computers, etc.
- is safely protected from air current fall out of
  dangerous radioactive isotopes released by military
  weapons being used in other parts of the world.

This lifestyle would seem quite improbable to attain
and live in the 21st century, so it's safe to say people
today do not have an adequate systemic defense against
DNA damage.

No authoritative body has discussed the potential
hazards that hydrogen peroxide bleaching agents contribute to the overall oxidative stress burden of the body
systems.

I personally feel that bleaching gels may play a very
significant role in tipping the degree of oxidative stress
within the body into an overwhelming toxic overload.
There is no doubt in my mind that if one's body is not
in perfect oxidant/antioxidant balance, then… whitening your teeth may lead to future health issues and a
reduced life span.

I also believe that, with good knowledge and strategy,
you can safely use hydrogen peroxide bleaching to actually benefit and improve your health. This is why I will

describe to you later how I supplement my body with antioxidants when I whiten my teeth with hydrogen peroxide. Now you know the "why," and you'll soon see the "how."

Before I reveal my "safer and more natural" way to whiten teeth, I would like you to know exactly why and how teeth stain. How do toxic substances enter the tooth? What is a detox and can you detox teeth?

You'll be surprised and shocked to learn about...

THE RAINBOW OF SMILES

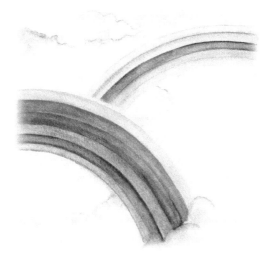

The Teeth Whitening Cure

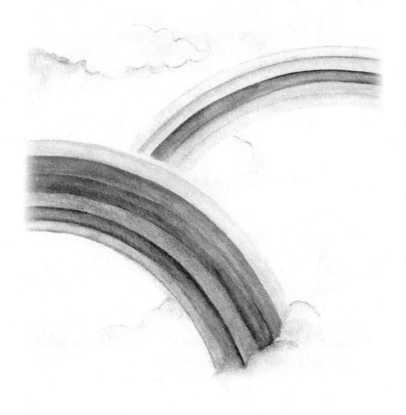

Chapter 13

The Rainbow of Smiles

The Rainbow of Smiles is a long chapter; therefore to make it easier for you to read and fully appreciate, I'm dividing it into two parts:

Part One... The Colors of the Enamel and Dentin

Part Two... The Texture of the Enamel Surface

When we look at a tooth's color and brightness, we see a composite of:

- the colors of the enamel and dentin,
- the texture of the enamel surface,
- the skin tone of the lips and face,
- and the sensitivity of the eye of the beholder.

Part One
The Colors of the Enamel and Dentin

The first protective outer layer of a tooth is called enamel, and it is sort of white. Enamel is considered the hardest substance in the human body. Usually enamel is the last part of the body to decay under normal burial conditions. The hardness and resistance of enamel to decay and trauma are why teeth are used to identify burn, crash, and explosion victims.

The next layer of tooth structure just below enamel is called dentin. The dentin is a yellow material. Both dentin and enamel are porous so that materials from the inner central pulp blood vessels and nerve can permeate it. Food and drinks that we ingest can also permeate through the outer enamel surface and change the natural color. As we get older, this flow of chromogenic material will accumulate into the tooth structure, and... cause it to darken to a brownish yellow. This happens because the enamel layer is translucent, and the color of chromogenic material within enamel, plus other structures that underlie it, tend to show through.

Because teeth enamel and dentin are porous, tooth discoloration is caused by the permeation of multiple "inside or intrinsic" and "outside or extrinsic" conditions. Intrinsic stains arise from within the tooth. Extrinsic stains are located on the outer surface of the tooth.

Intrinsic conditions may be:
- *dental fillings*
- *certain dental conditions and cavities*
- *trauma with internal bleeding of the pulp tissue*
- *infections*
- *medications*
- *nutritional deficiencies*
- *anemia*
- *bleeding disorders*
- *complications of pregnancy*
- *embryonic maturation development or lack of it*
- *genetic defects and hereditary diseases*

Extrinsic conditions may be:
- *dental plaque and tartar*
- *foods and beverages*
- *tobacco*
- *color pigment producing bacteria*

- ✓ *metallic compounds*
- ✓ *topical medications in the form of rinses,
  gels, ointments, and poultices.*

You will often hear that the most common cause of extrinsic stain is poor oral hygiene. Dentists and tooth-paste manufacturers often say that most tooth stains are due to the inability to remove stain-producing materials and/or the inadequate cleaning and polishing actions of toothpaste cleaners. This gives them a strong 'marketing voice' to sell you their "improved and more effective" toothpaste or toothbrush. This isn't exactly true, and misleading statements like this earn these huge corporate giants millions of dollars.

The truth of the matter is that porous enamel tends to trap, and then... allow food and beverage stains to penetrate deeper into the tooth. If your teeth stain easily, you likely have excessively porous enamel. Take note that ancient civilizations were noted for their very white teeth compared to today's societies. These ancient people were born with healthier teeth in most respects than people today are, and their enamel was better formed, more dense, and less porous. People from ages ago were born genetically superior to you and I from healthier and stronger parents. They ate organic whole foods, drank pure hydrating beverages, breathed pollution free air, and enjoyed plenty of life giving sun-shine. Their teeth did not stain as easily as yours and mine do, and they did not need electro-sonic tooth-brushes with space age nano-toothpastes to clean their teeth.

Let's face it—we are born weak compared to past generations. Not only is our enamel weaker and more porous, but... we tend to abuse our teeth with all sorts of acids to make them even more porous. Our teeth stain like a 'white diaper on green grass.' As an example, the acids in canned sodas, fruit juices, sports and energy drinks, and wine create rough spots and grooves. These rough spots and grooves enable chemicals in other foods and beverages that cause staining, such as coffee, tea, and tomato paste, to penetrate deeper into the tooth.

If you were born 500 years ago into a conscious community, chances are that your teeth would be healthier, whiter, and not stain very easily. I could write another book to answer why teeth stain today, but that is not my intention. I'll just briefly summarize a few points on why your teeth might look like the rainbow of smiles.

Extrinsic Stains

+ Microscopic defects in the outer enamel surface are susceptible to the accumulation of stains from food, drinks, tobacco, etc.
+ Diminished salivary output due to obstructions, infections, radiation therapy, chemotherapy, and medications plays a major role in the staining of teeth. A copious flow of saliva is needed to physically remove the sticky food debris and plaque.
+ Chromogenic pigment-releasing bacteria living at the gum line cause black, green, orange, and brown stains on the surface of enamel.
+ Industrial metallic compounds interact with dental plaque to produce surface stains. Mercury and lead dust cause blue green stain; copper and nickel cause green stain; chromic acid fumes give orange stain;

iodine makes brown stain; iron, manganese, and silver may stain the teeth black.

+ Dental mouthwashes can cause staining. Peridex with chlorhexidine is a common rinse to control gum disease and may cause brown stains. Cetylpyridium chloride in Cepacol, Scope, and Crest Pro-Health can cause brown stains. Potassium permanganate mouthwash causes violet stains; stannous fluoride in dental products creates brown stains.

+ Doxycycline and Minocycline antibiotics cause green-blue-gray staining of teeth when they form insoluble salts with natural fluids within the gum pockets and/or bind to glycoproteins in dental plaque.

Intrinsic Stains

+ Tooth crown formation begins while the baby is growing in the mother's womb; therefore, the potential for extensive intrinsic discoloration of the primary baby teeth may be present throughout pregnancy. Infections and toxemia that the mother suffers from may discolor the maturing embryo's teeth.

+ Dental fillings most commonly cause intrinsic discoloration. Mercury silver amalgam restorations can generate corrosion products (e.g. silver sulfide), which leaves a gray-black color in the tooth,

+ Trauma and tooth infections to developing yet unerupted permanent teeth can disturb enamel formation in the underlying developing permanent tooth. This may result in enamel hypoplasia, which is visualized as a localized yellow opacity on the erupted tooth. Unerupted permanent front teeth incisors commonly are affected this way after intrusion injuries to baby front teeth in young children who fall on their faces.

+ Crown formation of the secondary permanent teeth occurs until the child is about 8 years old. Systemic postnatal infections (e.g. measles, chicken pox, streptococcal infections, scarlet fever) can also cause enamel hypoplasia. The resulting band-like discolorations on the tooth become extrinsic stains after tooth eruption.

+ Teeth have internal nerves and blood vessels. If these nerves and blood vessels are damaged due to trauma, as for example... a volleyball smash into the face... the resulting internal bleeding may make the tooth become darker. The hemorrhage causes iron sulfide deposits along the dentin tubules, which produce a bluish-black shadow.

+ If a type of antibiotic called tetracycline is given to pregnant women, or children whose teeth are still developing, the child's 'baby' or 'adult' teeth may form with a bright yellow or greenish tinge. After the tooth erupts, the color gradually changes to gray or red-brown. This is a result of exposure to sunlight and photo-oxidation of tetracycline in the dentin-enamel interface, which produces a red-purple degradation product.

+ Excessive fluoride ingestion leads to toxic fluorosis. An infant can accidentally swallow just a pea-sized drop of fluoridated toothpaste and suffer from poisonous fluoride toxicity. That's why the label on fluoridated toothpastes warns you to call the poison control center if your baby swallows ANY toothpaste. Of course we all know that babies swallow toothpaste because they can't control this reflex; so the best solution is never to give your child any fluoridated products, including toothpaste and water. Take into consideration... if an infant drinks just 12 ounces of fluoridated tap water... he/she is likely ingesting more fluoride in the water than is considered to be a 'safe' level.

In its mildest form, fluorosis appears as faint white lines or streaks on the enamel. Moderate fluorosis has more obvious opaque regions referred to as enamel mottling, whereas severe fluorosis appears with extensive mottling that readily chips and stains, leading to pitting and brown discoloration.

Today nearly all children have signs of fluoride poisoning in the enamel of their teeth. Many dentists accuse the American Dental Association for their complicit help in poisoning our public water supply with drugs such as fluoride.

+ Vitamins C and D, calcium, and phosphate are required for healthy tooth formation. Nutritional deficiencies in either the pregnant woman or her child can cause enamel hypoplasia, a deficient layering of enamel structure resulting in yellow opaque spots.

+ Sickle cell anemia, thalassemia, and other blood dyscrasias hemolytic diseases of the newborn can produce a jaundice-like yellow green tint on the tooth surface.

+ Genetic defects in enamel or dentin formation include amelogenesis imperfecta, dentinogenesis imperfecta, and dentinal dysplasia. These are hereditary diseases with a propensity for intrinsic tooth discoloration. These genetic defects cause various staining colors from yellow to orange to opaque white, brown, and different dark tints of discoloration.

Part Two
The Texture of the Enamel Surface

The texture of the enamel surface can reflect light differently and make the tooth look brighter or darker. This is based on the optical properties of teeth, enamel, and water under visible conditions. The human eye also imparts a color to a tooth because the eye is typically more sensitive to green and yellow light than to blue or red.

Enamel contains 7–10% water by volume as one of its normal constituents, and this water affects its ability both to absorb and to scatter light. The light that penetrates the surface of a tooth and enters it is refracted due to the fact that light travels faster in air than in water or in solid enamel minerals. Tooth color is determined by the paths of light inside the tooth and the way they reflect into our eyes.

The appearance of enamel surfaces is affected by the surface reflection of light. Subtle grooves and other surface's discrepancies cause diffuse scattering of light. The accumulation of water in voids within the enamel causes opacity. The more porous the enamel, the less it scatters short (blue) wavelengths of light. Eliminating voids in tooth enamel by polishing, dehydration, and bonding synthetic plastic coatings alters the short wavelength (blue) scatter of enamel, thereby reducing its transmission of yellow light. The more the enamel scatters blue light, the lighter it appears.

Perfectly formed enamel scatters blue light to a very high degree. This is critical if you want your baby to have white teeth. For your baby to have white teeth you, the mother, must be in perfect health. Enamel surface texture is highly dependent on the mother, and to a lesser extent the father, transferring this quality to her child.

Tooth color is determined mainly by yellow dentin, but... enamel plays a significant role in 'modifying' tooth color by scattering the shorter wavelengths in the visible blue range. Greater scatter and reflection of blue light causes the tooth to appear "lighter and brighter."

Today, due to the poor lifestyle we have chosen, it is rare to find anyone with perfectly formed enamel. We no longer eat organic whole healthy foods, drink pure water, breathe unpolluted air, exercise, and think good thoughts. Neither did most of our grandparents and parents. For several generations we have been becoming constitutionally weaker with more sickness, disease, and poorly formed body, mind, and teeth. These facts are why the process of teeth whitening has developed into a billion dollar business for the dental and toothpaste industry.

Today, what we consider "normal" enamel transmits yellow and red light from the dentin to the enamel surface. Perfectly formed enamel, however, as the ancient cultures most likely had, scattered blue light into a gorgeous white smile. There were few rainbow smiles in the healthy social communities of our radiant ancestors.

I emphasize "healthy," because, if you read history, you'll learn that for quite a long time-span the European culture lived a very unconscious, unhealthy lifestyle. Unfortunately, you wouldn't find very many white teeth in the cosmopolitan cities of Europe. Most Americans with European ancestry at the writing of this book have genetically inherited disfigured, teeth and traditions of poor oral preventive care.

At the beginning of this chapter I wrote:

When we look at a tooth's color and brightness, we see a composite of:

- the colors of the enamel and dentin,
- the texture of the enamel surface,
- the skin tone of the lips and face,
- and the sensitivity of the eye of the beholder.

I strongly recommend that you do not whiten your teeth until AFTER you have read chapter 21— AVOID 'Over-Whitening'!

In that chapter… you will learn how skin tone and eye sensitivity influences the color and brightness of your teeth. This is VITAL information to help you from over whitening your soon-to-be gorgeous smile. Please, slowly and carefully, read the facts about the damage you can cause through OVER whitening.

I believe you now have enough information to help you understand the next chapter, which reviews the different reasons for and ways of whitening teeth. You'll also learn what it means to detox, and… why I believe it is important to detox your teeth.

I would like to now introduce you to incredible…

…STAIN BUSTERS!

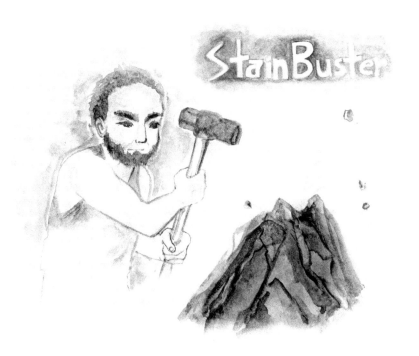

Chapter 14

...Stain Busters!

IF YOU'RE SPENDING TOO MUCH ON TEETH
   WHITENING...
IF YOU'RE LOOKING FOR A SAFER WAY TO
   BLEACH TEETH...
IF YOU'RE INTERESTED IN A MORE NATURAL
   LOOK...
I wrote this book for YOU!

It is understood that many people desire whiter
teeth. This is because they want a more attractive
smile and they want to feel more confident. A smile can
attract people and it brings the best out of people. However, many individuals do not smile because they do not
feel that their teeth are worth showing, especially in a
society where beauty has been categorized and labeled.
The concept of beauty nowadays has become ingrained
in the head instead of being spontaneous.

Simple observation of those around us quickly
reveals that the teeth of recent humans, collectively as
a race, display a wide range of different shades of white.
There is no one specific color that a person's teeth are
supposed to be, or should be. Some people's teeth are
just naturally lighter, or darker, in color than others.
All teeth do, however, have an inherent baseline color.
Lightening the baseline color of a person's teeth may be
a difficult task to achieve. Attempting to whiten teeth to
an unnatural level of whiteness can be expected to fail.

Even your dentist will not be able to unconditionally guarantee that you will be pleased with the outcome of your teeth whitening efforts. This is because many people have a very unrealistic idea of what constitutes a natural shade for teeth.

Some people will compare the color of their teeth to those people they see featured in films, on TV, or in magazine advertisements. In fact, the shade of many models and actors' teeth fall into the realm of "unnatural." The extreme shade you see has either been achieved by a means other than by bleaching (such as by placing dental crowns or porcelain veneers) or else never existed at all and instead was created by doctoring a picture.

Tooth color varies from person to person—just like skin and hair color. As we age the permanent teeth normally become more gray yellow, and darker. This age-related phenomenon is due to a progressive loss in translucent enamel from tooth wear that reveals the natural yellow color of underlying dentin. The thickness of a tooth's enamel becomes thinner revealing more of the darker dentin that lies underneath. The color of the dentin also tends to change over time. The technical dental terms for this natural wear due to aging are attrition, abrasion, erosion, and secondary reparative dentin.

A great deal of what we see as tooth color results from the play of light as it passes through the tooth's translucent enamel outer layer and then reflects back out once it has struck the opaque yellow inner dentin that lies underneath. Any circumstances, such as aging, that alters the properties of these tissues will have an effect on the color of the teeth.

The Teeth Whitening Cure

There are a number of ways that teeth can be made to look whiter if they become discolored. Some methods need to be professionally administered by a dentist, but most can be done right at home. This has been proven by myself and the whole Brighte-Smythe family.

Staining of teeth results from extrinsic and/or intrinsic staining. Extrinsic staining arises as a result of compounds such as tannins and polyphenolic compounds, which become trapped in and tightly bound to the proteinaceous acquired pellicle layer on the surface of the teeth. This type of staining can usually be removed by mechanical methods of tooth cleaning such as brushes, rotating rubber cups and tips, abrasive rubbing and polishing powders, pastes, soaps, sonic cleaners, magnetic water picks, and ionic inductive charges.

In contrast, intrinsic staining occurs when staining compounds penetrate the enamel and even into the dentin or arise from sources within the tooth pulp nerve and blood tissue. This type of staining is not amenable to mechanical methods of tooth cleaning. Chemical methods are required, including hydrogen peroxide in its many formulations, acids, bases, and chlorine bleach.

The color of teeth comes from genetics originally, and it varies person to person. If you were fortunate to be born of healthy parents with perfectly formed dense enamel, then your teeth would not stain easily. Unfortunately, our most recent ancestors have been losing their health and their perfect tooth structure due to lifestyle choices. Add to this the current standard of living most of us have chosen resulting in poor food selections, the lack of good nutrition in fast food restaurants, our polluted environment, negative thinking, and loss of spiritual connection, it should come as no wonder to us... as a result, our teeth stain fast and furious. The best way to keep teeth as white and bright as they were 'designed' to be have, is to avoid foods, liquids, drugs, and products that stain teeth. Remember that any food or beverage able to stain a white t-shirt, can ALSO stain your teeth.

The following information on how to clean teeth stains using home remedies is readily available on the Internet. You might find this interesting, and perhaps even try a few to see how well they work to remove your stains. I know through common sense and science what works and what is just hopeful dreaming, but within my family we have tested all these methods. Most of the Internet methods address extrinsic stains, but if you really want whiter teeth, you have to penetrate deeper into the enamel.

More importantly, I am only interested in "detoxing" my teeth to achieve radiant health, and... a 'gorgeous' smile. I'm not whitening them to look like a white refrigerator door. I am detoxing them in a safe, natural way to get more vibrant overall health while rebuilding my tooth structure into a more resilient and protective 'tiger like' snarl. I do not want an empty eggshell white look. I'm regenerating my teeth into a long lasting, beautiful, 'pearl like' smile.

Enjoy the rest of this chapter, and after you fall asleep from boredom, I'll electrify you with the way I detox and whiten my MY teeth. See you soon!

Stain Busters

A. Rub your teeth stains with the inner part of a banana peel or an orange peel.
B. Use the tip of your finger to rub off stains using any of these powders:
  - Neem powder
  - Walnut tree bark ash
  - Egg shell powder
  - Bamboo silica ash
  - Burnt toast
C. Brush your teeth with any of these oils:
  - Olive
  - Coconut
  - Sesame
D. Make these mixtures and brush your teeth with them:
  - vinegar + salt + baking soda
  - baking soda + peroxide
E. Brush your teeth with tooth soap such as pure olive oil Castille soap.
F. Chew and eat teeth cleansing, crunchy foods. The friction helps get debris off the teeth. some of these foods are:
  - Apples
  - Celery
  - Pears
  - Carrots
  - Broccoli
  - Cucumbers
  - Strawberries
G. This natural mixture works because of the malic acid it contains, which acts as an astringent to remove some of the surface discoloration on your

teeth. Though this method is perfectly safe to use on occasion, don't use it too often (no more than once a week) because the acid could potentially damage your tooth enamel.

Crush one ripe strawberry and mix with 1/2 teaspoon of baking soda.

Spread the mixture onto your teeth and leave on for five minutes.

Brush your teeth with toothpaste and rinse.

H. Brush your teeth as usual. Next, take your toothbrush, dip it into baking soda, then put a drop of lemon juice on it and brush your teeth. Rinse with water.

I. Each time after brushing your teeth just gargle with a small cap-full of peroxide, concentrating it on your teeth (don't swallow), spit out the peroxide and rinse with water.

J. Every time you brush, add baking soda to your toothpaste.

K. Gather ashes from a fire (a wood fire) and dip a wet toothbrush into the soot. Simply brush with the soot. Brush with toothpaste after to get the minty taste. The Crystals in the ash really make your teeth whiter right away!

L. Take some foil and fold it to form to your teeth. Take a little toothpaste and baking soda and mix together really well. Put some of the mixture into the foil and press and form it onto your teeth. Leave on for one hour everyday. Brush teeth normally afterwards.

M. Take a tablespoon of coconut oil and "work" it in the mouth by pushing, pulling, and sucking it through the teeth. The oil picks up dirt and grime leaving your teeth whiter.

N., O., P., Q., R., S., T., U., V., W., X., Y., Z., ...etc... all these methods work to some small degree but if you are really serious about whitening your teeth at home in a safer, more natural way, that may also increase your health and longevity then...

Don't Just Dump One of the Above Stain Busters, DUMP 'EM ALL! and Let's....

...DO DA DETOX!

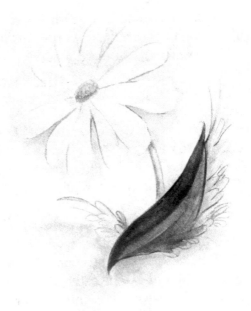

Chapter 15

...Do Da Detox!

The oral cavity including teeth and gums plays a critical role in the health and maintenance of the entire person. In order to contribute to the healing of the person as a whole and one's ability to maintain a proper level of health... I believe we should look to a more holistic evaluation of the procedures and therapeutic strategies of teeth bleaching practiced in dentistry.

Teeth are dynamic and alive. They are constantly building up and breaking down as they bite, chew, and grind. The daily stresses of wear and tear create an amazing amount of waste products. Yes, your pearly whites are living organisms and need to "sweat" in order to expel their metabolic wastes. If 'sweating' is interfered with or does not occur at all... the teeth cannot expel wastes properly, and this leads to more toxic teeth over time.

All through the ages of time humans have placed high value on proper daily exercise. Whether that exercise was in the form of work or play, sweat was always the end result. Sweat is one of the main pathways for the body to rid itself of accumulated toxins. Along with exercise came the sweat lodge, wet and dry heat sauna, sun ceremony, infrared sauna, hot and spicy herbal teas, skin brushing and slapping, and mortification of the flesh by flagellation.

Teeth are alive! Fluid flows through the tooth. Your teeth must sweat in order to cleanse the toxins they accumulate. "Sweat" is another word for "detox" which I will use from here on. Teeth detox internally through the pulp blood and nerve tissues. They also detox externally through enamel.

Surprise!

The byproducts of dental plaque are toxic poisons that contribute to decay, gum disease, and inflammatory processes in other organs of the body. Plaque forms waterproof covers on our teeth that allows the acidic—producing bacteria (strep mutans) to produce increasing concentrations of acid under these plaque covers. The more plaque, the more and larger the covers. This acid plays a role in dissolving the enamel layer of the tooth. These acid byproducts can also penetrate the tooth, enter the body's circulatory system through the pulp blood vessels, and burden the blood's pH stabilizing system. The tooth nerve is also challenged by plaque acids, and these nerves are connected to your brain. Now you can imagine how much harder your entire body, including your brain, has to work to cope with the stress of dental plaque.

If you want healthy, clean, and whiter teeth...

If you want a high performance athletic body...

If you want stronger organ function...

If you want a more efficient immune system...

If you want a clearer thinking brain...

IF YOU WANT A LONGER LIFE SPAN...

then you have to...

- detox the plaque off the surface of the tooth.

- slay the bacteria contributing to extrinsic stains.
- bleach out internal toxic stains, chemicals, resin and metal tags, and degradation byproducts.
- detox poisonous substances from inside the tooth through the pulp tissue.

Each day, we are surrounded by poisonous substances, which affect our minds and bodies. These poisonous substances are called toxins and your health is affected... much more than you may realize... depending upon how much exposure you have to toxins on a regular basis.

First of all, it's important to recognize that toxins can be found externally (outside your body and teeth) or created internally (inside your body and teeth).

Examples of external toxins are: pollution, second hand cigarette smoke, pesticides, artificial preservatives, hormones and antibiotics in food, and... vaccines.

Internal toxins, on the other hand, include bacteria and yeast that create dangerous toxins right inside your body. A low-grade, chronic viral infection, chronic stress, anxiety, or negative thinking, excessive exercise, over eating, fasting, anger, and excessive laughter produce internal toxins. And yes, even your thoughts and emotions are a source of internal toxicity!

The five major sources of toxins are:
Food
Water
Environment
Beauty and Personal Care Products
Stress and Negative Thinking
There are so many toxins in the environment that it is virtually impossible to eliminate or avoid them all.

There are over 90,000 industrial chemicals in our world environment. We know that there are over 200 chemical pollutants in embryonic cord blood. We are also now discovering pharmaceutical drugs in our tap water. Some of the most common drugs found in water are: antibiotics, anti-depressants, birth control pills, seizure medication, cancer treatments, pain killers, tranquilizers, and cholesterol-lowering compounds.

Most, if not all, of these toxins have potent oxidation activity in our body creating slow or quick poisoning and disease from excessive free radical burdens. The body's innate antioxidant system is not capable of protecting against all toxins, so it stores the overload in various organs, pigmentation, and inside teeth. The body needs help through nutritional vitamin and herbal supplementation plus regular detoxification to eliminate these toxins.

I bleach and whiten my teeth in a way that also detoxifies my teeth and body. My discovery is based on Chinese and Ayurvedic medical concepts that have identified a feedback loop/meridian system beginning in the mouth and ending in the Pelvic and Reproductive Organs. Today, new Allopathic Paridigms prove that tooth pulp, dentin, and periodontal ligament relate with the functioning of the heart, lymphatics, connective tissue, bone, kidneys, spleen, vascular/glandular systems, reproductive organs, and parts of the brain.

In agreement with Traditional Medical Concepts, the New Paradigm also shows that the tooth enamel is related to the skin, nails, hair, nerve tissue, and also parts of the brain that are susceptible to emotional conflicts. That is why tooth decay is high in children, teens, and pregnant women when emotional stress is higher.

When I bleach and whiten my teeth, I do it in a way which also detoxes the contaminated tooth structures such as enamel and dentin. Through the use of my method I am contributing to a whole body detox of accumulated toxic waste because of the relation of the mouth, teeth, enamel, and dentin with the various organs and tissue systems of the body. I am not only enhancing my smile, but I'm also advancing my life span and am giving myself many extra years of incredible radiant health and happiness.

When I look in the mirror and see stained teeth, I correlate this with accumulated toxic wastes that induce aging and degenerative disease. When I see my teeth become cleaner and brighter, I visualize my organs as cleaner, more youthful, and healthier. Cleaner, brighter, teeth = LESS body burden of toxic substances. When my teeth feel smooth and slick, I know that my total body energy flow is smoother. My "chi" or "prana" has less obstruction resulting in a healthier 'well-being'. I see the meridian systems connected with my teeth; I visualize every organ and tissue related with my mouth and teeth improving in function and vitality.

> **Detoxing teeth might be a difficult concept to grab at first, so let's review exactly what happens during bleaching.**

The majority of professionally monitored at-home teeth-bleaching compositions act by oxidation. The most commonly used oxidative compositions contain the hydrogen peroxide precursor carbamide peroxide, which is mixed with an anhydrous or low-water content, hygroscopic viscous carrier containing glycerin and/or propylene glycol and/or polyethylene glycol. Carbamide peroxide, also called urea peroxide, urea hydrogen peroxide, and percarbamide, is an oxidising agent, consisting of hydrogen peroxide compounded with urea. When contacted by water, carbamide peroxide dissociates into urea and hydrogen peroxide.

Adverse effects related with professional bleaching in addition to that of tooth sensitivity include:

• solubilization of calcium from the enamel layer with associated demineralization.

• penetration of the intact enamel and dentin by the bleaching agents, so as to reach the pulp chamber of a vital tooth thereby risking damage to pulpal tissue

• dilution of the bleaching compositions with saliva with resulting leaching from the dental tray and subsequent swallowing and digestion.

In summary, here are the important words connected with bleach gel:

— **Oxidation** creates free radicals, which could overburden the body's defenses.

— **Hydrogen Peroxide** burns soft tissue, proteins, etc. It is inevitable that during bleaching treatments some whitener will be swallowed. When whitener is swallowed it can cause irritation of the mucosal tissues of the mouth, lips, gums, palate, tonsils, tongue, and throat.

— Carbamide Peroxide is a generic pharmaceutical drug that is not found naturally in the body. It is not recommended for use in CHILDREN younger than 12 years of age except under the advice of a doctor. PREGNANCY and BREAST-FEEDING: It is unknown if Carbamide Peroxide can cause harm to the fetus. If you become pregnant while using Carbamide Peroxide, discuss with your doctor the benefits and risks of using Carbamide Peroxide during pregnancy. It is unknown if Carbamide Peroxide is excreted in breast milk. If you are or will be breast-feeding while you are using Carbamide Peroxide, check with your doctor or pharmacist to discuss the risks to your baby.

— Glycerin is a natural substance found in the body and appears to be relatively safe; however, it does have to be metabolized by the liver, and what is not excreted is stored as glycogen. Glycerin occurs naturally in fats and other substances, which are in part made up of lipid complexes. Glycerin may be derived from natural sources, primarily triglycerides, or be synthesized by the hydrogenolysis of carbohydrate materials or from products such as propylene. *Certain butanetriols can be contaminants of glycerin produced by hydrogenolysis of carbohydrates.* Evidence is available to show that glycerin is metabolized in the body to form glycogen or provide a direct energy source. In addition, long-term studies are available to show that synthetically derived glycerines are biologically similar to naturally derived glycerin.

If you are a bodybuilder, try this recipe before your next contest. The night before the contest mix up 1 cup of red wine and 50 ml of glycerin and sip this before going to bed. This helps to fill out the muscles. Glycerin temporarily draws water inside the muscle cells making them fuller. I guess now we'll see more bodybuilders bleaching their teeth. Might as well "pump up" the teeth along with muscles.

— Propylene Glycol is metabolized into lactic acid, which can burden the body's normal pH levels. It is also used to create artificial smoke or fog used in fire-fighting training.

Polyethylene glycol (PEG) is a chemical found in numerous products such as: laxatives, cosmetics, foods, drugs, body armor, tattoos, spandex, foam, paintball fill, gene therapy, etc. It is recognized by the FDA as having low toxicity. Some scientists, however, disagree, and claim that PEG is moderately toxic, an eye irritant, and a possible carcinogen. Many glycols produce severe acidosis, central nervous system damage, and congestion. PEG can cause convulsions, mutations, and surface EEG changes.

— Urea is, of course, found in urine and is in essence a waste product. It can be commercially produced, and I need not say more about this other than there is a popular therapy called Urine Therapy. For thousands of years, practitioners of urine therapy have believed human urine to have many preventative and curative powers. Some of the earliest human cultures used urine as a medicine. The urea in bleach gel is commercially made. In a manner of speaking, bleaching gel could be considered a health food. I would advise against swallowing this toxic cocktail.

— Enamel demineralization, damage to pulpal tissue, and swallowing with digestion are more problems

associated with teeth bleach ingredients. Demineralization is erosion of the enamel. It involves breaking up
the enamel calcium phosphate into calcium, phosphate,
and hydroxyl ions. Long term studies have not been
done to show possible damage to pulpal tissue, and
swallowing the bleach gel can lead to sore throat.
— Dental bleach gel releases mercury from mercury/
silver amalgam fillings. **Mercury** is one of the most toxic
substances known to man.
— Bleaching treatments increase the porosity of the
enamel. Excessive use of bleaching treatments increases
the loss of protein in enamel with possible permanent
long-term damage.
— In the presence of water hydrogen peroxide peroxide oxidizes or breaks down trapped colored pigments
within the teeth and changes them into colorless
byproducts. This produces the lightening effect. The
enamel and dentin of the teeth have water within their
structure, so the peroxide travels through the lattice
structure of the tooth penetrating deep in doing its job.
One has to wonder how the tooth eliminates the waste
of the broken down colored pigments.
— **Sensitivity** is the most common side effect of professionally dispensed, and... over the counter teeth
whitening products. In fact, data suggest that up to
75% of teeth whitening patients may experience unwel-
come sensitivity. Peroxide goes through the enamel and
dentin to the pulp in 5 to 15 minutes and changes the
genetic color of the dentin and the enamel as well as
removes stains. Sensitivity occurs when the chemical
by-products of carbamide and hydrogen peroxide pass
through the enamel-dentin layer and into the delicate

pulp nerve tissue. Research shows that as many as 40% of dental professionals recommend patients discontinue whitening procedures to alleviate related sensitivity.

— UV Light enhanced teeth bleaching may be dangerous to the eyes and skin. Studies show that the UV light damages skin and eyes up to four times as much as sunbathing.

— Conventional cosmetic dentists usually recommend that you brush your teeth with various fluoridated toothpastes to reduce sensitivity. Many of these toothpastes have these ingredients:

> **Fluoride**... highly toxic, poisonous, and carcinogenic.

> **Sodium Lauryl Sulfate**... a detergent irritating to soft tissues of the mouth. SLS leaves a soapy 'teeth film' which interferes with the innate natural remineralization of enamel. **Saccharin, preservatives, animal/artificial ingredients, color, and flavor**... all add to the toxic burden of the body.

All of the above information describes just a small drop of the negative toxic effects you would encounter when you whiten your teeth according to conventional methods. All bleaching is potentially dangerous, so I believe you must prepare yourself with the right information and means to protect yourself from accumulated toxic wastes during the whitening process. Adjusting your mind set from bleaching to detoxing might be a good start to turning a probable negative experience into a possible positive and beneficial life enhancing, self healing therapy.

After reviewing the literature, I have come to the conclusion that conventional teeth whitening and bleaching as practiced by many cosmetic dentists in the United Sates may have insidious harmful consequences. Each ingredient when examined alone may seem harmless, but... when mixed into a cocktail of bleach gel, I believe the ingredients as a whole contribute to a dangerous body burden of toxicity.

While we are surrounded by toxins, you can still feel and look your best by making better choices in the dental products you use. I believe my way of whitening my teeth is a better choice. It includes detoxifying my teeth, body, and mind. When you reduce your exposure to toxins, your body will actually feel better. A teeth detox takes away a huge burden on your liver and other organs of detoxification. When you feel the results of detoxing the waste from your teeth, you'll understand how all the organs and every cell of your body regain a more youthful beauty and vigor. A clean, detoxed, tooth is a healthier tooth. You will soon learn exactly how I whiten, and... detox my teeth.

Now I want to show you life saving...

...BASIC SELF DEFENSE

Self Defense

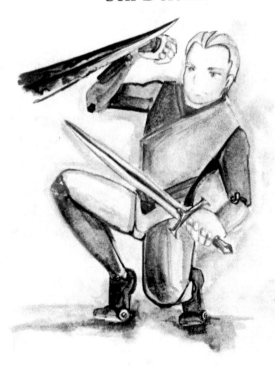

Chapter 16

...Basic Self Defense

The Brighte-Smythe family has been living a purist lifestyle ever since I met Jake at a raw food social brunch. I was just beginning my journey into a more natural lifestyle. Jake had years earlier discovered the benefits of organic foods while following the dietary recommendations of the Price-Pottenger Nutrition Foundation.

I have learned from and owe much to Jake for helping me integrate optimal health into my life. He's one significant force behind my success in the organic cacao confectionery trade. With his 'behind the scenes' guidance I have learned the secret to success. My passion is to empower others to achieve optimal health through dietary lifestyle changes including chocolate. Organic cacao is the super-antioxidant food that I provide to health-conscious individuals. One of my many rewards has been increased financial wealth.

Unfortunately, today most of the world has poorly formed and/or demineralized porous enamel. It sucks up brown cacao stains like the outer shell of a painted Easter egg. Writing this book about a teeth detox that also whitens and brightens chocolate stains has been most satisfying. Keeping my smile stain free has never been easier. I want the world to have this same luxury. I am driven to share with you all my research and experience with teeth detox whitening.

At this time let me bring more light onto the topic of hazardous toxins in general. Let's see what we can do 'beyond' bleaching, Let's find out how we can actually eliminate deep-seated stains and blemishes from within the tissues of our body. Let's learn how to purify our bodies of toxic waste. We now have at our fingertips thousands of years of knowledge and experience that can lead us to a more blissful life on earth.

———

Ancient cultures with excellent health employed a diet of unprocessed foods enabling them to maintain their teeth, bones, and resistance to disease. Dental decay was virtually nonexistent. Teeth color and brightness was retained for most of their lives. When groups within these cultures shifted to a diet including refined foods, sugar, and white flour, they 'paid a price' for this convenience... tooth decay, malformed dental arches, overlapping teeth, less resistance to disease, and discoloration of their tooth enamel.

My basic formula to protect myself from the toxic byproducts of teeth whitening begins with reducing my exposure to toxins in general. I start by adjusting my lifestyle to a more harmonious natural way, free of toxins, and as close as possible to the way my ancient ancestors lived.

The 5 most common sources of toxins today are:

Food
Water
Environment
Beauty and personal care products
Stress and negative thinking

Food... I choose whole foods that are, if possible, organic. This way I avoid some of the one billion pounds of pesticides used on food in the U.S. Basically I avoid foods that are packaged with a label of ingredients. If there is an ingredient label, then you can usually be assured that the ingredients have been man-made or tampered with in some way.

Water... I drink filtered and distilled water, and I use a shower filter to trap hazardous chlorine gases released during hot showers. I also avoid plastic water bottles and drinking/storage cups because of the toxins that leach from them. I avoid fluoridated water at all costs, because from my research I have discovered that no chemical causes as much cancer (and does this faster) than fluoride. Since I had been drinking city tap water 'enhanced' with fluoride for the first 30 years of my life, I am now supplementing my diet with Calcium, Magnesium, Phosphorous, and Iodine... experts have informed me that these minerals are the antidote for fluoride toxicity.

Environment... I try to use all natural cleaning products at home and have an air purifier to help reduce allergy contaminants and dust.

Beauty and personal care products... Anything put on the skin is absorbed into the body; therefore, I read the label on all cosmetics to determine their ingredients, thus enabling me to choose carefully which ones I would want to have within me. I usually opt for natural ingredients rather than man made chemicals.

Stress and negative thinking... The Centers for Disease Control and Prevention (CDC) estimates that up to 90% of all illness and disease is due to stress. I constantly read books and articles on how to live a more balanced stress-free life. Everyday I practice stress relief through the use of mental and physical exercises.

This covers Basic Self Defense and should help prepare you for the onslaught of toxic waste and free radicals during teeth whitening sessions. If you have years of accumulated toxins and tissue damage, as I do, then you may need additional cleansing by water fasting, vegetable juicing, and sweat therapy. I engage in each of these practices, plus oxygen therapy and colon cleansing.

Water Fasting... Water fasting is an ancient method. The digestive system is given a rest from breaking down food. The extra energy available goes toward eliminating waste from the body. I water fast one 24 hour day per week.

Vegetable Juicing... Once per month I water fast for 3 days. I will add some vegetable juices to restore energy that I need for my daily activities. The green juices also help detoxify the blood and liver.

Sweat Therapy... The skin is the largest organ of the body. Toxins are absorbed and eliminated through this protective barrier. Because time and money are involved in some sweat therapies such as dry / wet/ infrared heat saunas, sweat lodge, and others, I keep it simple using daily physical exercise to work up a sweat.

Oxygen Therapy... 6 minutes without oxygen could result in either death or brain damage. This is one reason we should improve our oxygen utilization. Another serious reason is that oxidation efficiency = cellular energy production. Your mitochondria converts oxygen to water plus energy. This chemical process creates free radicals. If your mitochondria become dysfunctional, then you will have decreased free radical buffering antioxidants. This means you will have increased free radical formation... resulting in you retaining less energy, aging more rapidly, and becoming diseased. The better your mitochondria process oxygen, the longer you will live.

Decrease in oxygen efficiency usually begins in the 30's age group. It is characterized by not enough oxygen in the blood stream, inflammation, toxicity and infections, stress, nutritional deficiency, hormonal deficiency, and decreased fitness. Oxidation therapies are designed to increase efficient utilization of oxygen. Most oxidative therapies need to be supervised by a physician. There are some simple home remedies which I will mention, but due to the sensitive nature of this information, you will have to research the methods yourself. Ozone therapy, oral hydrogen peroxide, exercise with oxygen therapy (EWOT), interval training, Buddhist meditation, Qi Gong exercise, Yoga, and Tai Chi are several therapies that I use periodically at home.

How permeable your tooth structure is to oxygen is one of the main determinants of how white and how quickly your teeth will respond to teeth bleaching. Your teeth can be rejuvenated to their youthful ability to absorb oxygen. I do everything possible to make certain every cell in my body, including teeth, utilizes oxygen with peak efficiency.

Colon Cleansing... There is a saying, "all disease starts in the mouth, but death begins in the colon." The road to health begins with intestinal cleansing and detoxification. The intestine is one of the main 'drain-pipes' to eliminate toxic waste. If you want to detox your teeth, the colon has to be in good working order.

Colonic irrigation is popular with many natural health care practitioners; however, it is not one of my favorite therapies. I have tried it and prefer to use herbs with slower results. My approach is to use prebiotics, probiotics, vegetable fibers, and chia seed. The important herbs used are marshmallow root, licorice root, bitter gourd, black walnut hulls, slippery elm bark, pumpkin seed, cascara sagrada. Yoga can also help tonify the intestinal muscles for peristalsis and more thorough elimination.

More specialized therapies that I use are:
- Replacing mercury silver fillings with porcelain/resin tooth colored fillings.
- Supplements that bind with toxic metals.
- Chelation with suppository formula.
- Vitamins, herbs, and supplements that neutralize free radicals.
- Vitamins and Herbs that facilitate teeth sweating.
- Oil Pulling.
- Tongue Rolling and Teeth Tapping.

Replacing mercury silver fillings... There is NO Safe Filling Material. Every artificial man made tooth filling has some level of body burden and toxicity. Mercury in silver amalgam fillings, however, is currently the most toxic, and I recommend replacing them when you feel the time is right. It is better to use fillings and crowns that have a minimum of metal. There appears to be more bio-field energy interference with metal constructed into and over teeth.

———

Supplements that bind with toxic metals... Modified citrus pectin, sodium alginate, zeolites, chlorella, cilantro, and bentonite clay are supplements that bind with and excrete toxic metals such as mercury, lead, arsenic, cadmium, and nickel.

———

Chelation with suppository formula... Chelation is another way to trap and excrete toxic heavy metals. "Medicardium EDTA" is the suppository brand that I use. Because most heavy metals are excreted through the feces, one has to be sure the colon is functioning well, or the metals will linger in the colon and get reabsorbed into the blood stream.

Vitamins, herbs, and supplements that neutralize free radicals... Antioxidants help the body manage excess free radicals.

• Glutathione is the body's innate natural and most important antioxidant.

• Vitamin C is the major water soluble antioxidant found in plants. Because it does not occur naturally in the body, we have to eat foods plentiful with "C" or supplement with it.

• Vitamin E is a fat-soluble antioxidant.

• OSR#1 is one of the latest antioxidants developed by a biochemist. It is one of the few antioxidants able to cross lipid cell membranes especially into the mitochondria power-house of the cell. OSR#1 scavenges free radicals and helps maintain healthy levels of glutathione. It is a new supplement and is getting close but guarded attention from the natural health care community.

• Herbs that support antioxidant activity are Reishi Mushroom, Lycium Fruit, Dioscoria Root, Ginkgo Root, and Curcuma Root.

Medical University studies showed that various combinations of herbs and supplements protected brain cells in vitro. When cultured human brain cells were oxidized with H_2O_2 for 3 hours, pretreatment with herbal mixtures doubled the number of surviving cells.

———

Vitamins and Herbs that facilitate teeth sweating... In order for a tooth to sweat it needs clean blood vessels and efficient heart pump action. Regular exercise is important to maintain flexibility and open flow of the venous/arterial highway. Certain exercises develop resistance to impact to help protect the body. All exercise initiates critical lymph flow. Pumping lymph through the body is nature's miracle pipeline to excreting toxic waste.

• **Clean Blood Vessels**
Vitamin B Family is the most basic group for heart health. B-12, 9, & 6 help remove homocysteine from the blood. High levels of homocysteine can cause artery damage. B-3 improves flexibility and oxygen transport and reduces cholesterol plaque formation.

There is well-established evidence suggesting that

Enzymes dissolve scar tissue and plaque within blood vessels. Popular ones are nattokinase, lumbrokinase, serrapeptase, and other proteolytic enzymes. Fermented natto soybeans and dairy cheeses have gobs of natural enzymes.

- Efficient Heart
Padma Basic is my favorite of the many herbs that improve heart function and circulation. It has been clinically researched in Switzerland to eliminate the symptoms of chronic tooth pulpitis (sensitivity) and even prevent root canals by increasing blood flow to the roots of teeth. I don't know of any other herb complex that can make this claim. I use it daily.

- Exercise
The only way to move lymph is by gravity and exercise. Toxic waste is primarily moved through the lymph. If you are bleaching teeth, lymph movement is essential. Inversion exercise such as toe touching and head stands, where the heart moves below the level of the hips, is very common in yoga. These movements use gravity to move the toxic waste though the lymphatic tissues.

- Tongue rolling and teeth tapping
Are Chinese exercises that work the muscles, ligaments, and lymph around the face, jaw, and teeth. Every Qi Gong teacher knows these exercises, so you would have no trouble learning. Tongue rolling stimulates salivary function which is important for the exchange of minerals and waste between the enamel, dentin, and pulp tissue. It also energetically moves

115

the chi within and around the teeth to increase vital function.

Teeth Tapping vibrates the hard yet supple tooth structure and associated fluids setting up shock waves that help push the toxic waste out. Teeth tapping also strengthens the tooth structure against the impact of daily biting, chewing, and grinding. Human enamel is brittle. Like glass, it cracks easily; but unlike glass, enamel is able to contain cracks and remain intact for most individuals' lifetimes. The major reason why teeth do not break apart is due to the presence of tufts— small, crack-like defects found deep in the tooth at the dentin-enamel junction. Acting together, these tufted cracks suppress major tooth chips and fractures due to trauma and biting by distributing the forces amongst themselves.

Enamel also has "basket weave" micro structure which protects against crack growth. Teeth have a self-healing process where organic material fills cracks extending from the tufts. This type of infilling bonds opposing crack walls and increases the amount of force needed to break the tooth. Teeth tapping uses this unique self healing feature of cracking, healing, cracking, healing... to rebuild and strengthen teeth. Martial Artists make use of this natural crack-heal training to rebuild and strengthen their body so that they can break baseball bats with their shin bones, or bricks with their hands and heads. You should be able to achieve similar results with teeth tapping. A healthy tooth should easily crack walnuts and other hard shell foods. Find a Qi Gong teacher to show you how.

As you can see, it is vital that teeth sweat and breathe adequate oxygen in order to pump and exchange fluids, minerals, and organic substances with the oral cavity and inner circulatory system. I do everything possible to make my teeth sweat.

- Oil Pulling

There is no question that the body can be healed through oral cleansing. Science has proven there are many links between oral health and degenerative disease. Oil Pulling is an ancient method of oral cleansing that originated from Ayurvedic medicine. Some claim it is one of the most powerful and effective methods of detoxification in natural medicine. A tablespoon of oil, such as coconut oil, is worked in the mouth by pushing, pulling, and sucking it through the teeth for about 15–20 minutes. The oil sucks up toxins, bacteria, and pus. You then spit out the dirty oil and brush your teeth clean. I oil pull occasionally and do believe the method works well for sucking up waste from the gums, but my teeth do not turn as white from this practice as many practitioners claim.

Basic Self Defense is an enormous subject of study, and I cannot give enough attention to it in this book about teeth whitening.

Now that we have discussed Basic Self Defense I would like to give you a few...

...WORDS OF CAUTION!

The Teeth Whitening Cure

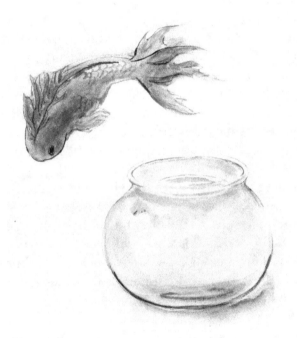

Chapter 17

...Words of Caution!

What I am revealing to you is knowledge that Dr. Q. gained through much research with trial and error. They don't teach this in dental school. She had to search for thousands of hours and spend a small fortune of her income to come to this realization. If 30 years ago I had known the information I'm sharing with you now, I would not need to bleach my teeth today. I wish I had started detoxing my teeth and body way back then.

Results Vary from Person to Person

It's important to bear in mind that bleaching doesn't always result in the whiteness that you expect. The results vary from person to person and depend on the shade of your teeth before bleaching. The whitening effects of different bleaching methods can last for a few years, but this varies from person to person. Research on dentist-prescribed "home" bleaching treatment has found that for people who achieved a lighter shade, only half of them still had whiter teeth six months later. Your eating, drinking, smoking, and brushing habits may have an effect on how long the treatment lasts.

Radioactive Carbon-14

Since bleaching my way is also a teeth detox program, I usually detox my teeth at least every 6 months. I have accumulated a lot of toxic waste over the years, and it takes time to eliminate it in a slow, safe, and comfortable manner.

I have to offer one comment on what a teeth detox can and cannot achieve. The aboveground nuclear tests that occurred in several countries including the United States between 1955 and 1963 dramatically increased the amount of radioactive carbon-14 in the atmosphere and subsequently in the biosphere. People world-wide were contaminated with this isotope and it became measurable in the tooth enamel. After the tests ended, the atmospheric concentration of the isotope began to decrease. I'm not sure if my teeth detox can eliminate this radioactive isotope from your teeth. There is, however, a positive effect of this discharge of radioactivity into the biosphere.

One side effect of the change in atmospheric carbon-14 is that this enables a special instrument to determine your birth year, because the amount of carbon-14 in tooth enamel can be measured with accelerator mass spectrometry and compared to records of past atmospheric carbon-14 concentrations. Since teeth are formed at a specific age and do not exchange carbon thereafter, this method allows age to be determined to within 1.6 years. However, this method only works for individuals born after 1943, and it must be known whether the individual was born in the Northern or the Southern Hemisphere.

Unpredictable

The results home teeth whitening can produce are not always easy to predict. At any one point in peoples' lives the color of their teeth can and will be influenced by a number of different factors. Most certainly some types of tooth discoloration are more resistant to lightening than others. Teeth detox, however, is always predictable. Some degree of teeth detox always occurs when you follow your program.

Not Simple

Unlike teeth detox (a very simple procedure), teeth bleaching is not just a simple cosmetic operation. At some point you should have your dentist diagnose the cause of the staining or discoloration to establish a prognosis of whether the stain can be removed or not. Mild fluorosis from toxic ingestion of excess fluoride has a white appearance, because there is altered mineralization at the site. The changes in mineralization cause an increased deposition of water in the enamel, which changes the refractive index of the tooth and alters the natural scatter of light. Severe enamel fluorosis is more difficult to bleach.

Will Not Lighten Dental Work

Some tooth discolorations are associated with existing dental work. Before bleaching is performed, defective restorations should be replaced. As a general rule, teeth whitening treatments cannot be expected to lighten existing dental work.

May Need Root Canal

A tooth that has been traumatized, such as having been bumped in an accident, may change color. In this case the darkening of the tooth can be an indication that there is a problem with the health of the nerve inside the tooth. For this reason any individually darkened tooth should always be evaluated by a dentist. It may need a root canal treatment. Teeth that have had root canal treatment often need whitening. It is common knowledge that a tooth that has had root canal treatment will darken over time.

I am still concerned with the safety and effectiveness of today's root canal treatments. A high percentage of them never completely heal. They continue to harbor chronic toxic disease-spreading bacteria. This chronic toxemia is one infection the body is not able to tolerate. The bacteremia float like toxic sludge from the tooth root into various susceptible sites within the body tissues. Our vital organs—heart, lungs, liver, kidney, spleen, brain, etc. are an especially serious end point, which may lead to degeneration.

Even root canals that appear successful have a tendency to crack irreparably some years after therapy.

But don't panic. Fortunately, with the advent of advanced laser disinfection, we may be near a resolution for root canal bacteremia. Root canal treachery has been with us for over one hundred years. If you are heading for a root canal, buy yourself time and find a dentist who is well-experienced with laser technology.

I know a few people who were told they needed root canals for chronic tooth sensitivity and pain. They tried the herb, Padma Basic, to buy time to make decisions. Their symptoms disappeared, and several years passed without a root canal.

Doctors and dentists often don't have all the answers. Their knowledge is limited to the training they get in medical and dental school. Very few western-trained medical professionals are open to traditional herbs, supplements, and healing therapies. New paradigms of health are being discovered in the alternative healing world. Open up your mind and heart to the world of possibilities; a world that looks beyond cutting, burning, and drugging as healing tools. Tomorrow's healing may be as beautiful as clouds floating in the sky and rivers meandering through valleys.

See Your Orthodontist

After orthodontic treatment it is common for small residues of bonding resin to remain on the teeth after the removal of brackets. This lowers the reflectivity of the surface enamel. The bleach will not penetrate the residue-bonding agent, and it has to be professionally removed before bleaching.

Maximum Whiteness

All teeth do not reach the same whiteness; each tooth has its maximum whiteness beyond which it will not whiten, regardless of the technique or material. Teeth among different people do not bleach at the same rate. Some will bleach faster than others. Once the rate of the shade change is exceeded, higher concentrations of peroxides make no difference in the color change. Excessive bleaching, however, can make the teeth appear abnormal.

Ghost Teeth

Especially nowadays people tend to see beauty in white teeth. Bleaching does have a beautiful effect, but it is not without side effects. Sometimes, in an attempt to achieve an unnatural shade of tooth whiteness, a person will exceed the treatment recommendations. This type of whitener abuse can put the person at risk. Bleaching treatments increase the porosity of the enamel. Excessive use of bleaching treatments will cause a loss of protein in enamel and therefore increases the water content making the enamel become more opaque. This will make the enamel optically abnormal. It can lose its pleasing, natural, and warm glow. You might end up with a ghostly bluish appearance.

Sensitivity

Prolonged exposure of teeth to bleaching hydrogen peroxide could cause unwanted and uncomfortable sensitivity. Remember that hydrogen peroxide oxidizes interprismatic extrinsic staining within tooth enamel. Tooth sensitivity is believed to result from the movement of fluid through the dentinal tubes toward nerve endings in the tooth. This movement is enhanced in typical bleach gels by the carriers for the carbamide peroxide. In fact, it has been determined that glycerin, propylene glycol, and polyethylene glycol can each give rise to varying amounts of tooth sensitivity following exposure of the teeth to heat, cold, and overly sweet substances. I do not use carriers in my bleaching method so this simplifies dealing with side effects.

Demineralization

Demineralization of enamel is one of the more common reasons why your teeth might be unusually sensitive to hydrogen peroxide. Tooth enamel is composed almost entirely of calcium phosphate $(Ca_5 (PO_4)_3 OH)$. The chemical process of the formation of enamel is called mineralization. It is a combination of calcium, phosphate, and hydroxyl ions. The reverse process is called demineralization. An acid medium will favor the process of demineralization. An alkaline medium will favor the process of mineralization. Healthy saliva will provide just the kind of medium which will favor the process of mineralization, both on account of its neutral or slightly alkaline character and the calcium and phosphate ions it can provide.

Eating Disorders

If you have a low resting salivary pH, the enamel can dissolve into the oral fluids. As a result, the exposed dentin lacks a protective layer. Gastric reflux disease, eating disorders where the person vomits, citric fruit juices, soft drinks, sports/energy drinks, worn and chipped teeth, and cavities also result in extensive loss of tooth mineral and tooth structure. An indication of overeating and poor digestion is a dry mouth or lack of saliva. This leaves the mouth unprotected and prone to demineralization and tooth decay. This result is open tubules in the dentin, which makes the teeth very sensitive to the oral environment as you eat, drink, breathe, and when you apply hydrogen peroxide.

Pregnancy

During pregnancy hormonal changes result in a dramatic decrease in the buffering capacity of the saliva. Reduced protection from saliva combined with frequent acid challenges due to morning sickness nausea puts pregnant women at a high risk of demineralization. Occupation-related dehydration along with high daily intake of carbonated cola drinks can also lead to salivary acidification and related enamel demineralization. I do not recommend teeth bleaching when you are pregnant. I certainly don't recommend any type of detox for the body or teeth if you are pregnant, or trying to become pregnant, without first consulting with your personal physician.

Medical Conditions

Medical conditions such as diabetes mellitus, Sjorgen's syndrome, and chemical drug medications can lead to salivary dysfunction resulting in enamel and root surface demineralization. An acidic oral environment allows the overgrowth of cavity-forming bacteria. Cavities will be hypersensitive to hydrogen peroxide. Sores in the mouth will also be very sensitive to certain concentrations of hydrogen peroxide.

Poor Diet

A poor diet and digestion leads to slightly acid saliva—an environment which accelerates demineralization of enamel. Healthy saliva is neutral or slightly alkaline and is not conducive for harmful bacteria, which needs an acid medium to do damage. Demineralized enamel is becoming a world-wide epidemic.

It is generally thought that tooth enamel that has been demineralized and eroded is lost forever. The hard enamel and the dentin covering the tooth may appear inert, but this is a misconception. Living cells have built these structures. When the body is in need of calcium, demineralization takes place. This means that during calcium deficiency, the body can rob the enamel and dentin, as well as bones, of calcium. If demineralization is possible during calcium deficiency, it is reasonable to assume that remineralization can take place when there is an adequate supply of calcium and other favorable conditions. A good diet and eating habits are essential for remineralizing and maintaining healthy teeth, gums, and bone.

Teeth are alive! Fluid flows through the teeth. When you have decay, the fluid flows from the mouth, into the enamel, through the dentin, and into the pulp nerve. If you use conventional bleach gels when you have a cavity, the bleach agent goes through the tooth into the nerve pulp and starts killing the pulp. A thorough examination by your dentist will give you the condition of the current health of your mouth. This should help you decide if you should practice home bleaching or not. Teeth detox, however, because of its slow cautious approach is relatively safe, unless you are pregnant or suffer from a serious life-threatening disease, in which case you should always consult with your physician.

Now we can ask the question...

...SHOULD I OR SHOULDN'T I?

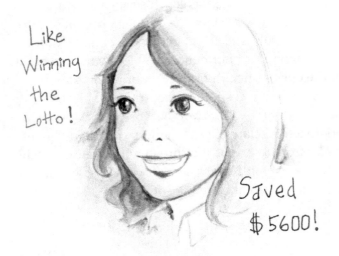

Chapter 18

...Should I or Shouldn't I?

The only question remaining is, "should I whiten my teeth with professionally dispensed bleach gel and/or over the counter whitening products?" or "should I lighten my teeth with a teeth detox?"

At the time of writing this book the typical cost of basic professional in-office teeth whitening with take home trays is around $150.00–$400.00 per arch. This translates into $300–$800 to whiten both the top and bottom teeth. Laser whitening and/or UV lights run about $1200 for a one-hour session. Deep Bleaching with adjunct services, such as micro abrasion and specialized enamel surface preparation that alters light reflectivity, can approach $1800.

The Brighte-Smythe family saved $5600 by incorporating the teeth detox into their lives. That was an easy "should I?" for us.

The laser and UV light treatment gives absolutely no benefit over bleaching without UV and may damage skin and eyes up to four times as much as sunbathing. Studies have shown that one week after bleaching there was no significant difference in efficacy between those teeth bleached with UV irradiation and those bleached without irradiation. It has long been known that heat from bleaching lamps may cause temporary additional dehydration of the enamel, which results in an immediate increased whitening effect. Also realize... after a couple of days of re-hydration, bleaching procedures with or without lamps have similar lightening effects.

Aggressive 'dentist-controlled' bleaching also exposes more grooves on the enamel surface of bleached teeth as compared to unbleached teeth. These grooves make the teeth more vulnerable to mechanical stress.

Some researchers note that teeth typically can restore their previous hardness after losing small amounts of enamel calcification. They conclude that human enamel has been shown to heal itself and remineralize over time. This means it has the ability to restore back the levels of surface calcium that has been lost due to bleaching.

However... other laboratory studies suggest that teeth bleaching products for home use may minimally reduce the surface hardness of tooth enamel and enamel's ability to bounce back from normal wear and tear.

Dr. Q personally feels that the faster and more aggressively one tries to bleach teeth, the more difficult it is to restore the calcium levels of the enamel. In her opinion, a teeth detox is slower, safer, and more comfortable than dentist-prescribed systems. It should be easier to restore and remineralize the enamel when you detox teeth.

I personally can state that the slower, safer, teeth detox eliminated a number of prior sensitive areas on my teeth. I attribute this to the better remineralization that occurs when using the more natural products in the detox.

Studies have shown that often less than 50 percent of the whitener is present in the dentist-administered take-home trays one hour after application. The amount of leakage may be even higher in over-the-counter whitening products, in which the trays are not custom-fitted by a dentist. Your saliva mixes with this leakage, and then you end up swallowing and digesting it. In my opinion, your health may be at risk if you ignore the possible hazards of free radical body burden that comes with all bleaching methods.

Teeth detoxing and lightening at home costs pennies—plus you benefit from the whole body detox program you choose, which may include vitamins, herbs, supplements, mental and physical exercise, etc. The eventual outcome of whitening is the same regardless of the material if the time is extended long enough, as the outcome is determined by the tooth... not the product. However, you will never get a teeth detox with conventional bleach gel systems.

In my opinion, there are many questions to ask about the safety of 'dentist-administered' and 'over-the-counter' teeth whitening systems. After weighing the pros and cons, I choose to detox my teeth and bask in a gorgeous, radiant, healthy, and uplifting experience. So do my family, friends, and business associates.

Before revealing to you my total teeth detox, I would like to introduce you to...

...THE STAIN SLAYERS

The Teeth Whitening Cure

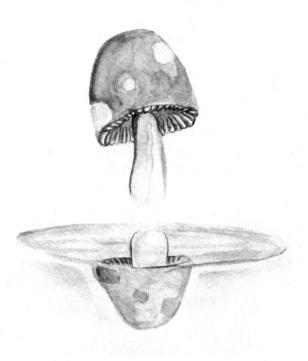

Chapter 19

...Products to SLAY Teeth Stains

Over the years Dr. Q discovered a variety of Stain Slayers. These products are not widely known to the public. She uses them because they are superior to what you find at the stores.

Most importantly, she and I both Avoid All Toxic Fluoride Toothpastes sold at most stores. Health-conscious dentists rarely use fluoridated toothpaste to clean their patients' teeth, because they know they are dangerously toxic and don't work well. They certainly don't use any fluoridated products, including water, for themselves and family members. Holistic dentists also use special formulations that don't include sodium lauryl sulfate(SLS). SLS is found in most over-the-counter toothpastes. Manufacturers include this chemical in their toothpaste, because consumers seem to like the foamy texture it creates. The foam is a big selling feature. So, of course, in order to sell more toothpaste and compete in the marketplace, 99.99% of toothpaste manufacturers include it.

Unfortunately, what the buyer doesn't know is that SLS leaves a slimy, soapy residue on the teeth and gums, which actually prevents thorough cleansing of the enamel surface and inhibits natural breathing and oxygenating functions of teeth and gums. Tooth powders and soaps are the best way to clean teeth at home. One of my favorite tooth powders is MicroBrite. (HYPERLINK "http://www.thewolfeclinic.com/" http://www.thewolfeclinic.com/)

MicroBrite antioxidant tooth powder whitens my teeth without harsh abrasion for a brilliant smile and fresh mouth. MicroBrite has an antioxidant in it called Microhydrin, which raises the pH of the mouth to a healthy alkalinity while neutralizing mouth acids. This helps fight tartar, gum inflammation such as gingivitis, and tooth decay.

MicroBrite also has Xylitol and Aloe. Xylitol inhibits plaque by lowering plaque/enamel surface tension. Aloe is a medicinal plant containing anti-inflammatory agents to soothe and promote healing of oral tissues.

Food particles that make up plaque have a positive ionic charge. MicroBrite releases negative hydrogen ion electrons, which can help neutralize the positive charge of plaque. This helps reduce the surface tension of these particles allowing them to lift, solubilize, and be removed with a toothbrush. I get an amazing burst of antioxidant stain busting foam penetrating every nook and cranny around my teeth and gums. Leaves my mouth sparkling clean and fresh.

MicroBrite is also very pure in that it contains NONE of the following found in most toothpastes:

Fluoride... highly toxic, poisonous, and carcinogenic.

Sodium Lauryl Sulfate... a detergent irritating to soft tissues of the mouth. Leaves a soapy film on the teeth that prevents natural minerals in saliva from healing enamel defects. Saccharin, preservatives, animal/artificial ingredients, color, and flavor... all add to the toxic burden of the body.

Tooth Soap is another excellent cleaning agent. Unlike conventional tooth cleansing products that coat the teeth and gums with contaminating ingredients, Tooth Soap® cleaned teeth facilitate re-mineralization from nutrients in the diet/saliva. Gums are also encouraged to strengthen with the nutritional oils in tooth soap. (HYPERLINK "http://www.toothsoap.com/" http://www.toothsoap.com/)

Coral Calcium and Bentonite Clay are all natural mild abrasive powders that I brush my teeth with. Because of their abrasive nature I usually use them only on the days that I bleach my teeth in order to prepare the enamel surface for better penetration of the bleaching agent. Both are mild abrasives and also natural supplements that you can actually swallow. That is exactly what I do—I swallow my tooth-powder after brushing in order to take advantage of the health supporting properties it offers. [Coral Legend / Medi-Clay from http://HYPERLINK "http://www.prlabs.com/" http://www.prlabs.com/

I would never dare do that with conventional store-bought fluoride toothpaste. In fact, if you check the label on your toothpaste tube you will see this FDA WARNING:

"If you accidentally swallow more than used for brushing, seek professional help or contact a poison control center immediately."

There is a reason for this warning. There are toxic, poisonous chemicals in any toothpaste that has this warning. My natural tooth powders are perfectly safe to ingest. In fact they not only protect and support my teeth and gums but also are whole-body nutritional supplements with outstanding health benefits.

Coral Calcium is 100% Japanese Sango Marine Coral Concentrate Powder. It is composed of highly ionized calcium, magnesium, and trace minerals, which help promote an optimal alkaline tissue pH. Coral Calcium is especially useful for bones, teeth, and joints. All forms of calcium must be ionized via your digestion before they can be absorbed. Since coral minerals are already highly ionized, they are easily absorbed (even by the elderly and those with poor digestion).

Coral Calcium has legendary effects for rapidly promoting an alkaline pH for whole body health and vitality. It is also an excellent powder for brushing off tooth stains, but... use it sparingly and occasionally due to its abrasive nature.

Most people are already familiar with the benefits of calcium—magnesium minerals in Coral Calcium, so I'm going to highlight Bentonite Clay.

Calcium Bentonite Clay has a history of being used extensively by many cultures for thousands of years. In natural medicine it has been used for prevention and curing problems such as toxicity, parasites, and infections. It is said to bind to free radicals, raise red blood cell count, strengthen immunity, and stimulate cellular respiration. It has detoxifying properties, which trap waste products thereby improving liver function, digestion, and elimination.

Bentonite clay carries a uniquely strong negative ionic charge, which causes it to attract magnetically any substance with a positive ionic charge (i.e., bacteria, toxins, metals, etc.). These substances are both adsorbed (sticking to the outside like Velcro) and absorbed (drawn inside) by the clay molecules. Your body does not digest clay, so the clay passes through your system collecting the toxins and removing them as the clay is eliminated. This is another reason to colon cleanse and keep your digestive system healthy and moving.

The clay's immediate action upon the body is directly on the digestive channel. This involves the clay actually binding with the toxic substances and removing them from the body with the stool. It performs this job with every kind of toxin, including those from the environment and those that occur naturally as by-products of the body's own health processes. The clay and the adsorbed toxins are both eliminated together. This keeps the toxins from being reabsorbed into the bloodstream.

Bentonite Clay has a cumulative negative charge when hydrated, and scavenges mostly positively-charged ions and toxins such as heavy metals and bacterial food plaque that form on teeth, thus neutralizing them. There is research currently in progress studying this 'life saving' clay in battle-ground wound care and destroying flesh-eating bacteria.

Today our diets are mineral-deficient. Bentonite Clay consists of no less than 67 necessary minerals found in all tissues and fluids and taking part in all body processes. They include calcium, magnesium, zinc, iron, silica, manganese, boron, bromide, as well as other macro and micro-elements.

I vary the daily use of my tooth brushing products according to the foods and herbs that I eat and drink. Some herbs stain teeth heavily, so I'll brush with Coral Calcium mixed with Calcium Bentonite Clay on the days I drink these herbs. Other days when I fast I'll "dry brush," which means brushing my teeth with a plain dry conventional toothbrush. Other days I'll use my ionic toothbrush without any powder or soap. Another day I might use Tooth Soap in the morning and Micro-Brite in the evening.

DentiCal is an ionic solution of magnesium, calcium, and ascorbic acid (vitamin C, untreated by heat).
The solution is synergistic in creating and protecting
the healthy appearance of cells of the teeth and gums.
Ionic absorption of calcium, magnesium, and ascorbic
acid into the jaw, teeth, and gums is the key element
design for DentiCal. Sometimes I'll dip my ionic toothbrush into Dentical or just rinse with it after brushing.
Ingredients: Steam distilled water, two special-formula
highly-charged ionic calciums synergistically bound,
magnesium, real lime juice, colloidal silver, raspberry
flavor. (HYPERLINK http://www.GlobalLight.net www.
GlobalLight.net)

Orgono Living Silica is a little-known dietary supplement which is coming of age.

Traditionally, natural silica from the Indian bamboo
tree was used to rebuild enamel and bone structure. As
early as 1878 Louis Pasteur predicted that silica would
be found to be an important therapeutic substance
for many diseases and would play a significant role in
human health and consequently nutrition. We now
know that silica is absolutely essential for the body to
create and maintain collagen. Collagen is an important
part of the tooth enamel-dentin matrix that gives it
toughness and flexibility.

Some of the places you need silica are:

Connective tissue strengthening and support (joint,
ligaments and muscles).

Bone strengthening and support through enhanced
calcium absorption.

Strengthening of teeth and gums.

Cardiovascular support for supple arteries and veins and in removing plaque from artery walls.

Healthy skin tissue. The skin is our first line of defense against pathogens.

Prevent thinning hair, brittle nails, and dry skin.

Silica has been shown to be a good eliminator of aluminum. Aluminum has been implicated as a cause of Alzheimer's.

As we age, scientific measurements have shown that the human body retains less and less silica. The average American diet does not contain adequate levels of essential nutrients, especially silica. It is primarily found in natural oats, millet, barley, wheat, and potatoes. If we eat these foods at all, they are normally refined to a point where all the silica has been removed.

A unique example of the power of silica is seen in special Marine Glass Sponges, which are unusual skeleton structures. They are defined as natural silica-based nanostructured composite materials. There is a specific sponge species that synthesizes the largest biosilica structures on earth. They are noted for their pencil-sized rod spicules having a combination of properties of toughness combined with stiffness and resilience. One can take a pencil-sized rod spicule of a meter or more in length and bend it into a circle without breaking it. When the load is released, the spicule recovers its original shape. This same property of silica with its tough, fibrous nature gives teeth their longevity.

Orgono Living Silica is the most naturally sourced and processed bio-available silica on the market. I swish and drink an ounce nearly everyday. (HYPERLINK "http://www.sunfood.com/" http://www.sunfood.com/)

The Teeth Whitening Cure

Quinton Marine Plasma (QMP) is seawater collected from specific regions of the vortex of plankton blooms. It is diluted to the correct tonicity to be the closest composition match to the natural internal environment of the human body. The product evolved from the hypothesis on the evolutionary progression of uni-cellular life in the sea to multi-cellular life on the land. It has 100+ years of a proven track record in correcting and supporting the establishment of the optimum internal environment of the body. The internal environment of the body is the mainstay of health... with disease being the result of adverse changes within this ideal environment.

Since 1904, Quinton Marine Plasma has proven to be the optimum medium to support correct homeostatic function. Indeed Quinton himself described it as "the origin of life." He confirmed this in a series of daring experiments on dogs. His ultimate proof was where he drained a dog of all blood to the point of no palpebral reflex and replaced the removed blood volume with QMP. Not only did the dog survive, but upon recovering was more active and healthy than before.

Alexis Carrell, 1912 Nobel Laureate for Physiology and Medicine, began an experiment that kept cells from an embryonic chicken heart functioning for 34 years. Eventually public outcry led to the termination of the experiment. His 'secret' was the use of Quinton's QMP as the daily cleansing and restoration fluid.

Dentists are using QMP to flush root canals, aid bone and soft tissue healing in the mouth, and improve mineralization of teeth. When I whiten my teeth I swish with QMP to help replace lost minerals from the enamel. During other time I swish and swallow 1/2 tablespoon weekly to help remineralize my teeth and to establish optimum internal homeostasis. (HYPERLINK "http://www.originalquinton.com/" http://www.original-quinton.com/)

The Ionic Toothbrush, the most innovative toothbrush of the future is here now and requires no toothpaste. Tooth enamel has a healthy negative anionic charge. Calcium, iron, bacterial plaque, and toothpaste have net positive cationic charges. Since positive and negative attract each other, the bacterial plaque biofilm, and stains attach to the tooth enamel.

The ionic toothbrush has an internal battery, which produces a direct current electric field via the bristles. This negative electric field induces a positive charge to the enamel surface. Since positive will repel positive, the ionic toothbrush initiates an immediate new field at the tooth interface that repels dental biofilm plaque and stains off the enamel. This is many times more efficient at cleansing the teeth than customary manual brushing.

In order to help prevent stains and cavities one has to remove infected plaque biofilm from tooth enamel. You might find it hard to believe, but it is nearly impossible to brush, floss, irrigate, pic, etc. dental plaque and stains from all tooth surfaces. This is especially true if your toothpaste is formulated with SLS.

If you believe that fluoride is a safe chemical that prevents cavities, and I do not, you will also be surprised to know that the fluoride in toothpaste generally does not penetrate through plaque onto the tooth enamel. The sodium fluoride (NaF) is concentrated mostly at the plaque/saliva interface. During the 30 to 120 seconds of brushing very little of the fluoride actually penetrates through plaque bio-films into the plaque/

enamel interface. This is why toothpaste companies and dentists always recommend brushing for 3 minutes, or 180 seconds, in order to break through the plaque into the enamel surface. As you know, very few people brush a full 3 minutes. The average time is 30 seconds. In 30 seconds very little, if any, fluoride penetrates through plaque to reach the enamel surface.

The next time you brush your teeth with your "miracle" fluoride toothpaste, say a prayer. Only a prayer answered could create the 30 second miracle of any effective fluoride permeating your tooth enamel.

The bristles on the ionic toothbrush are very soft and gentle. I use my regular toothbrush during the times I bleach my teeth with cleansing powders of coral calcium and bentonite clay. I use the ionic brush, at times dipped in Dentical, during maintenance phase. I use Microbrite antioxidant tooth powder and Tooth Soap on other days when I feel a need for an antioxidant boost. I'm constantly changing among different products depending on which foods and drinks I'm ingesting. (HYPERLINK "http://www.dentist.net/" http://www.dentist.net/)

Oratec Pocket Irrigator is a mini-pocket irrigator for irrigating periodontal pockets. About the size of a small eye drop bottle, it holds 2oz. of solution and is ideal for irrigating a few deep pockets, yet small enough to put in a purse or pocket if you travel. It's available in a wide variety of tip styles, one of which is sure to be exactly right for you.

If you are serious about detoxing your teeth, you should not ignore your gums. The Oratec Pocket Irrigator delivers antibacterial solutions under the gum line into deep gum pockets where gum disease bacteria colonize. This irrigator is the perfect carrier for 0.2% sodium hypochlorite and 3% hydrogen peroxide antibacterial solutions. It's like a mini "squirt gun on steroids" that kills germs in infected gum pockets to help fight gum disease. (HYPERLINK "https://www.oratec.net/" https://www.oratec.net/)

Pepsodent's White Now Toothpaste is not available in the United States at the time of writing this book, but it is available in Europe. I'm not in favor of using it. I know, however, that some of you are not convinced of the risks involved with conventional toothpaste ingredients. This may be just right for you during emergencies when you haven't had time to whiten your teeth.

Pepsodent's White Now Toothpaste has an instant whitening effect delivered immediately after brushing with its novel silica whitening ingredient containing blue covarine. A statistically significant reduction in tooth yellowness and improvement in tooth whiteness was measured immediately after brushing with blue covarine. Makeup for your teeth? Why not? But honestly, the effect will not last forever. When you brush your teeth with the White Now paste, your teeth will be covered with blue foam that includes the color ingredient Blue Covarine. The color sticks on your teeth but not on your gums. It's just like makeup—the color will stay there for a while and disappear later. The blue color makes yellowish teeth appear whiter. So it's just an optical illusion that will not stay, but who cares! So much cheaper than getting porcelain veneers or professional bleaching by dentist.

On one of our European vacations the girls experimented with White Now. They thought it was so "you know, happening." They had a lot of fun with instant whitening. At their age, they still think they are unbreakable, and the fluoride in the toothpaste didn't seem an issue. I let them experiment, but the White Now stayed in Europe when we returned home.

Finally... It is a good idea to have your teeth professionally cleaned by a dentist or dental hygienist to remove tartar and surface stains that regular toothbrushing cannot achieve. Bleaching agents will not penetrate hard calcium deposits and stubborn cigarette nicotine stains on the enamel surface. Plus your dentist can whiten and brighten your teeth by altering the light scattering properties of your enamel with simple polishing techniques. You may not need special bleaching gels to lighten your teeth, if lightening is all you are interested in. If, however, you are interested in detoxing your teeth, I do suggest you consider my teeth detox.

The clinical stages in teeth lightening are as follows.

• Normal tooth enamel has a lustrous smooth surface which reflects light. The light must be evenly reflected from the surface back to the eye in order to create a bright white sheen.

• Basically, a dentist or hygienist polishes and smooths the rough tooth surface, making it reflect more light and appear brighter.

• This can be followed by more gentle micro-abrasion using phosphoric acid etching and application of flour of pumice or graded abrasive pastes at low rotational speeds. Micro-abrasion with nano-silica increases the reflection of light and back-scatter of the shorter wavelengths of light to make the tooth appear even lighter. The etching step enhances subsequent subsurface mineral changes. Hydrogen Peroxide may then be applied to oxidize and bleach cellular chromophores to a colorless state.

• Sodium hypochlorite (chlorine bleach) may also be applied to dissolve organic matter further.

• The process may be repeated to reach deeper into the tooth.

Remember that a chromophore is part of a molecule responsible for its color. When the chromophore in the molecule absorbs certain wavelengths of visible light and transmits or reflects others, the molecule has a color. The chromophore has to be chemically altered to change the color. This is accomplished with acids, polishing agents, oxidation with hydrogen peroxide, and dissolving organic matter with sodium hypochlorite (household bleach). It is important to maximize the microscopic porosity of the enamel surface by etching combined with gentle abrasion. Etching with acid removes the surface pellicle and makes the superficial enamel more porous allowing ions to penetrate deeper into the subsurface region.

Realize... the eventual outcome of whitening is the same regardless of the material if the time is extended long enough, as the outcome is determined by the tooth not the product.

* Bleaching is not permanent *

– Teeth regress eventually to worse than what one started with if bleaching is stopped totally because the bleach makes our enamel more porous ...

– thus a cycle of bleaching and more porosity and tooth damage ...

145

– possibly more and more free radicals and DNA breakdown.

This is why you must !!!! !!!!

...follow by re-mineralization therapy to strengthen enamel that has been made more porous with acids.

When you perform a teeth detox correctly, you will eventually notice that it becomes easier to maintain the bright whiteness, because you are remineralizing the teeth from inside and outside. With time this should make the teeth less penetrable to toxic stains. Remineralizing also normalizes the scatter of light reflecting to your eyes. This optical property is the key to flashing a whiter, brighter smile.

I hope that I have successfully explained the benefits of including a teeth detox into your oral hygiene home care.

At this point you have enough basic information to begin preparing your body for a teeth detox by supplementing with vitamins, herbs, exercise, etc.

The next chapter will reveal to you the core application of my teeth detox, which is...

...WAY, WAY, DIFFERENT!

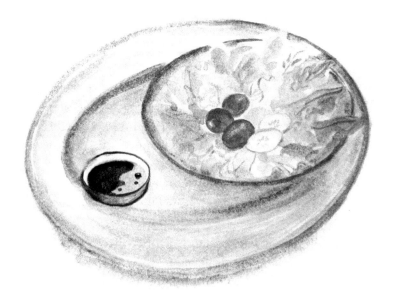

Chapter 20

...Way, Way, Different!

Braen did an Internet search for the world's longest living communities of people. He found that they tend to live relatively isolated from largely congested metropolitan areas. They live, work, and play hard in naturally clean and beautiful environments. They all also included super-antioxidant foods and herbs in their diet. The well-documented Hunza of Pakistan ate super-antioxidant apricots. The famous Okinawans, a fiercely independent race of people residing on the Island of Okinawa in the Ryukyu Islands southwest of Japan, ate the Ashitaba plant. Centenarians of Central Asia had the goji berry. Southern Chinese discovered the miracle grass gynostemma. Chinese that live beyond 100 years drink green tea. Superior health and supportive nutrition is a key player in maintaining the balance between oxidation and anti-oxidation. Unless we consume adequate antioxidants in our diet, oxidation will contribute to oxidative stress, chronic inflammation, and disease. It is generally agreed by the entire scientific community that oxidative stress is a major factor in most human diseases. Under conditions of elevated oxidative stress humans need to increase and expand their diet with antioxidant rich foods, herbs, and supplements to reduce free radical damage. A dietary program that contains a variety of antioxidants has been proven to double the in vitro life of brain cells after being exposed to oxidants.

If you are like most American living life on the "edge," then any disturbance to your balance of oxidants vs. antioxidants may cascade into an over inflated balloon of free radicals. You might then tip into a slow downward spiral of physical degeneration and reduced longevity. Chemical ingredients in teeth-bleaching gels, in my opinion, are biohazards that can overwhelm your body's innate ability to neutralize free radicals. I would like to add a couple more comments to this argument, leaving no stone unturned. I am driven to convince you of the value in supplementing with super-antioxidant foods, herbs, and vitamin supplements when you whiten your teeth. Even my safer and more natural method to whiten teeth creates free radicals, but... with proper nutritive support I feel that I can protect myself.

If you have already bleached your teeth in the past, then you might have experienced the "zing" sensitivity to cold afterwards. The "zing" which you interpret as sensitivity to cold is actually a result of the teeth drying out during the bleaching process. When we bleach teeth, the evaporation of oxygen produced from the hydrogen peroxide action dehydrates the teeth. That is why the teeth always look a little chalky right after bleaching. They have dried out, lost water content, altered light reflection, and look extra white and chalky. Without water in the enamel the light wavelengths do not scatter as much giving the teeth a whiter appearance. In other words they are dehydrated.

When you detox your teeth, you are really forcing them to "sweat" and clear out toxic substances. Bathing your teeth in hydrogen peroxide is like stepping into a hot humid sauna. They are going to sweat like your teeth have never sweat in your life. This will lead to some dehydration, which is good if done in a safe, controlled manner. Regular exercise, as you know, is very healthy, and a little dehydration is one very effective way to detox the teeth and body. When you lose water, the body responds by tapping water from deeper inner tissues and organs to replace the water lost at the surface. Toxic substances will be carried out and eliminated with the sweat. There is a safe limit, though, and if you dehydrate beyond this safety zone, then long-term damage may occur.

A dehydrated tooth is no different than a dehydrated body. It puts an enormous strain on the body to maintain homeostasis. Our bodies are about 70% water and every metabolic system depends on water to function at peak efficiency. Excessive "sweating" leads to dehydration and breakdown of cell tissue creating a huge amount of destructive free radicals. Stay dehydrated for too long and you will end up in the hospital hooked up to an I.V. Your veins will be sucking up sugar water to rehydrate and hopefully save your life. Dehydrating a tooth excessively won't put you in the hospital. However, if you dehydrate a tooth beyond its safety zone, it could send you to the dentist with a horrible toothache. Repeat this tooth abuse too often and free radicals accumulate. With time your tooth could die floating in a bag of free radical pus.

Here is a bonus piece of information I'm giving you. Very few people know this. Eating food is an example of a perfectly normal body process that can lead to free radical stress. Who would have thought?

I find this a perfect introduction to my 3 girls. I'm so proud of them!

Raw foods are extremely nutritive and supportive during a teeth detox. My 3 girls are expert chefs at creating raw food recipes. They keep their daddy's tummy well-satisfied and nourished during weekends when they help prepare meals. On the weekends all I do is provide the chocolate dessert—organic, of course.

♩ ♪ ♫ Love...Love...Love... ♭ ♫ ♪ ♫

I'm sure you eat salads and other tasty raw foods with oil and vinegar dressing. When you chew and grind your seasoned raw salad, there is a "mini-detox" occurring. The vinegar is an acidic medium, which dissolves grime-like plaque and bacterial colonies from your teeth and gums. The oil binds with and sucks up the loosened grime. You then swallow and the body takes in the accessible nutrition from food while it eliminates the grime through the intestinal tract.

Your teeth and mouth have just undergone a "mini-detox." Free radicals are involved in this miracle, which could lead to oxidative stress, if you are not in balance. This is much like the motor oil you put into your car engine. The motor oil picks up dirt and grime from the internal workings. When you drain your oil, the now "detoxed" engine is cleaner and ready to drive you another 5 thousand miles.

The lesson here?

When you detox your teeth—use nutritional support to prevent free radical stress.

I tend to believe alternative authorities who brought to light the dangers of Fluoride in our water and Mercury in our silver fillings. They are now saying that the polymers and monomers in tooth-colored composite fillings also have negative consequences. Let's face it. There is nothing man-made that is 100% safe to put into the mouth. There is no 'safe' filling material. Some of us have made mistakes, and some of our parents made mistakes, which led us to develop cavities in our teeth. We must make choices in filling materials to save our teeth, and so I choose the safest ones available at this time. Mercury silver fillings are the most dangerous of all. I had all mine replaced with white fillings. They all, however, in some way add toxic byproducts and burden our body with free radicals.

A teeth detox, in my opinion, is the best way to cleanse and restore my teeth and gums to their more natural state. This I hope will extend the life of my teeth and allow me to enjoy a long, healthy, vibrant life span. I want to glow with energy and radiance in every aspect of my life. I want a drop dead gorgeous smile... and my teeth detox gives me exactly that in a safer and more natural way.

In the next chapter I have a...

WARNING!
AVOID 'Over-Whitening'!

...Way, Way, Different!

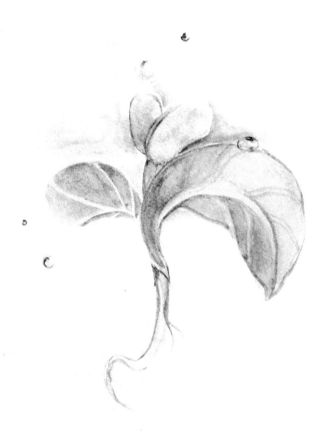

Chapter 21

AVOID 'Over-Whitening'!

In chapter 13, "The Rainbow of Smiles," I wrote:
When we look at a tooth's color and brightness we see this is a composite of:

- the colors of the enamel and dentin.
- the texture of the enamel surface.
- the skin tone of the lips and face.
- and the sensitivity of the eye of the beholder.

I warned you about over-whitening your soon-to-be gorgeous smile. I said it is critical to take into consideration skin tone and eye sensitivity. Here are the facts...

Studies have proven that the whitest smile is not always the prettiest. People were tested, and it has been found that we do not always favor the whitest smile. We also do not perceive all skin colors to be equally attractive with bright white teeth. Different colors and brightness of teeth were found to be prettier with a various combination of skin colors and tones.

This is why it is important to change the color of your teeth slowly and gradually. You want comment and feedback about your whitening process. You should have a close friend, relative, co-worker, mate, and lover give you their opinion on how they perceive the color of your teeth. Do they feel that the new color of your teeth is complimenting your skin color and tone? Should you go whiter or stay at the current level of brightness?

Remember, you admire your teeth twice a day when you brush them; first thing in the morning and last at night. The world judges your smile all day long. Your gorgeous smile might be the make or break first impression for success!

Be very cautious in this respect. If you bleach your teeth alone, without comment from your circle of friends, then there is the possibility of excessively bright white teeth that may be perceived by others as too bright depending on your skin color and tone.

The tooth detox is one of your best formulas for superior health. Follow the guidelines in this book and you'll also end up with a natural, luxurious, drop-dead-gorgeous smile.

Go slow and glow! I now award you with my sincerest...

Congratulations!

You are now ready to begin the Detox.

Chapter 22

The Detox Formula

Gather each of the following...
• Toothbrush with Soft Bristles
• Dental Floss
• Inter-proximal Plaque Removers (wood, plastic, or brushes) Coral Calcium and/or Calcium Bentonite Clay
• Clear and Colorless Acidic Beverage with about a 3.0pH; for example:
  ✓ Safeway Diet Tonic Water with Carbonated Water and Citric Acid
  ✓ Dry Soda: Juniper Berry with Carbonated Water and Phosphoric Acid from the Dry Soda Company
  ✓ Jones Pure Cane Soda: Cream Soda with Carbonated Water and Phosphoric Acid from the Jones Soda Company
  ✓ Seven-Up with Carbonated Water, Citric Acid, Potassium Citrate
  ✓ Sparkling White Wine: Carbonated, Clear, Colorless
• Cotton Tipped Swabs
• 2 Tongue Cleaners with Handle
• 1/2 or 1 ounce Glass Eye-Dropper Bottle
• 2 Glass or Plastic 16-ounce Empty Bottles
• 2 Glass or Plastic One-Ounce Shot-Glasses
• Rubber Gloves

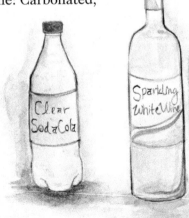

156

- Distilled Water
- Food Grade 35% Hydrogen Peroxide (HYPERLINK "http://www.pureh2o2forhealth.com/" www.pureh2o2-forhealth.com)
  - 5% Sodium Hypochlorite (e.g. household bleach)
  - Mineral Water Rinse (e.g. Quinton Marine Plasma)

Preparing the Formula

NEVER allow children to handle hydrogen peroxide.

35% H_2O_2 is extremely dangerous, and contact with skin will immediately cause skin to turn white due to oxidative burning. H_2O_2 is exceedingly hazardous if splashed into eyes, and… could cause permanent eye damage. You'll want to wear protective eye-wear during your preparation of the detox formula. It also may be lethal if swallowed. Be sure to follow instructions on the bottle in case of accidental contact on skin and/or eyes, or… upon swallowing. Always have copious amounts of water readily available when handling H_2O_2. Water is an antidote for H_2O_2. ALWAYS wear rubber gloves when handling 35% hydrogen peroxide.

Store hydrogen peroxide in the freezer.

H_2O_2 has a low freezing point and will not freeze in your typical home freezer. Hydrogen peroxide degrades with heat. Storing in the freezer will extend the life of the product.

24 hours prior to beginning the detox:

1. Prepare the Bentonite Clay per instructions on the bottle. Usually I mix about 1 teaspoon clay powder with 10 teaspoons distilled water in a small glass container and then let it hydrate on the kitchen counter overnight. It will turn into a sort of mud by the next day.

2. Fill the small eye-dropper bottle with 35% hydrogen peroxide. Use rubber gloves to prevent burns.

3. Pour 12 ounces distilled water into an empty 16-ounce bottle. Add one ounce 35% H_2O_2 to the bottle. This dilution makes about a 2.7% hydrogen peroxide solution, which is a little less than the concentration you would buy at your neighborhood store.

4. Label and store all 3 bottles of hydrogen peroxide in the freezer... 1 bottle 35% strength hydrogen peroxide... 1 bottle 3% strength hydrogen peroxide... 1 eye-dropper bottle of the 35% strength hydrogen peroxide. The eye-dropper bottle should always hold the 35% strength hydrogen peroxide.

5. Pour 12.5 ounces distilled water into the other empty 16-ounce bottle. Add 1/2 ounce 5% chlorine bleach to the bottle. This dilution makes about a 0.2% sodium hypochlorite solution with an 8.5pH. The solution is only good for 30 days because of natural degradation. A new, fresh dilution has to be prepared every 30 days.

Label and store in a cool dark place. Do not freeze!

Applying the Formula

At this point I'm confident that my body is saturated with free radical-neutralizing antioxidants. For at least

The Detox Formula

2 weeks prior to the detox I have been supplementing my diet with super-anti-oxidant herbs and supplements. During the next 2 weeks of detox I increase my anti-oxidant dose of vitamin C.

DAY ONE of the detox I lay out all my supplies.

(1) I make a small 1/4 teaspoon mixture of Bentonite Clay and Coral Calcium.

(2) I brush my teeth thoroughly with this paste and swallow after brushing to take advantage of the nutritional benefits of these two powders. Then I clean plaque from inter-proximal spaces using dental floss and other cleaners such as picks and brushes. I finish with a swish rinse of distilled water, which I drink to engage the health benefits of the calcium/clay/distilled water.

(3) I pour one ounce of 2.7% hydrogen peroxide into one of the shot-glasses.

(4) I pour one ounce of sodium hypochlorite into the other shot-glass.

(5) At this point I take one ounce of the acidic beverage of my choice (usually my preference is carbonated white wine), and swish my teeth with it for 60 seconds. After one minute of swishing I spit this out.

I look in the mirror to see how much of my upper teeth show when I smile. If I have a low smile line and my lips do not clear the entire tooth, then I use my tongue scrapers to lift up my lip above the upper teeth so they are all clearly exposed.

(6) I take a cotton tipped swab, soak it in the 2.7% H_2O_2 and dab the solution focusing on the upper front 6-10 teeth. I try to avoid the gums and lips. I keep soaking and dabbing (inside/outside surfaces) for 10 minutes.

It is relatively difficult to dab the back molars with H_2O_2. I concentrate on the 6 front teeth and the 4 side teeth bicuspids. These are the teeth that show when I smile. The rest of the teeth will detox by rinsing with 2.7% H_2O_2, 0.2% sodium hypochlorite, distilled water, and Quinton Marine Plasma as described in steps #7, 9, 10, 11, 12.

(7) After 10 minutes I pour the remaining 2.7% H_2O_2 from the shot-glass into my mouth and swish for 60 seconds. I spit this solution out.

(8) I take another cotton tipped swab and soak it in the other shot glass filled with sodium hypochlorite. I dab this solution on my teeth for 10 minutes.

(9) After 10 minutes of dabbing, I pour the remaining solution from the shot-glass into my mouth and swish for 60 seconds. I then spit this solution out.

(10) I rinse with distilled water and spit out.

(11) I drink 1/2 glass distilled water.

(12) I finish the day's detox by swishing my mouth for several minutes with Quinton Marine Plasma to remineralize the teeth. I then swallow this nourishing supplement.

I examine my gums in the mirror to see if there are any white spots visible which would mean I have gingivitis or inflamed tissue. Healthy gums should not burn with 3% H_2O_2. If there are white spots, then the oxygenating properties of hydrogen peroxide followed by sodium hypochlorite rinsing should help restore the tissue to a healthier state within a few days.

DAY TWO repeats as day one except I change the concentration of the dabbing H_2O_2.

If there are no visible white spots on the gums, then I increase the concentration of the H_2O_2. I use the eye-dropper and transfer 24 drops of distilled water into one shot-glass. I transfer 3 drops of 35% H_2O_2 into the same shot glass of distilled water.

After 10 minutes of dabbing with this stronger concentration I pour 2.7% H_2O_2 into the shot-glass, rinse with the 2.7% H_2O_2 for 60 seconds, spit out, and then... continue the protocol steps 1–12.

DAY THREE repeats as day 2 except I change the concentration of the dabbing H_2O_2.

If there are no visible white spots on the gums, then I increase the concentration of the H_2O_2. I use the eyedropper and transfer 24 drops of distilled water into one shot-glass. I transfer 4 drops of 35% H_2O_2 into the same shot glass of distilled water.

After 10 minutes of dabbing with this stronger concentration, I pour 2.7% H_2O_2 into the shot glass, rinse with the 2.7% H_2O_2 for 60 seconds, spit out, and again... continue the protocol steps 1–12.

DAY 4, 5, 6, etc. repeat except I change the concentration of the dabbing H_2O_2.

**Whenever white spots are visible on the gum tissue I do not increase the concentration of the H_2O_2. I continue daily detoxing at the same level until no more white spots occur. Only then do I increase the concentration of hydrogen peroxide by one drop each day. I never use a mixture greater than 17.5% H_2O_2. That means I never mix more than 12 drops of 35% H_2O_2 with 24 drops of distilled water.

If my teeth become sensitive to temperature changes while eating and drinking, then I stop the detox for a few days to allow recovery time. This is no different than when you get sore muscles from a work out. Recovery time is important for growth.

I noticed that as my gum tissue became healthier, it also became more resistant to higher concentrations of hydrogen peroxide. I believe this is similar to other extraordinary abilities that people develop. Consider those that can walk on hot coals, withstand burning desert sun, or meditate in the Himalayan mountains covered only with drenching wet bed sheets. It seems that the healthier one becomes, the stronger and more resistant one is to extreme variations in the environment.

Once I discover the strongest concentration of hydrogen peroxide that I can use without creating white spots, I continue detoxing at this level for 2 weeks. I believe it is reasonable to detox teeth at least twice a year

A Strong Word of CAUTION! on Hydrogen Peroxide

Pharmaceutical Grade 3% sold at your local drugstore or supermarket has a variety of stabilizers which I AVOID putting in my mouth. These stabilizers include acetanilide, phenol, sodium stanate, and tertrasodium phosphate.

Beauticians 6% grade is used to color hair. Reagent Grade for scientific experiments, Electronic Grade to clean electronics, and Technical Grade are 30-35% H_2O_2 and also have stabilizers and additives. They are NOT for oral use.

> # Food Grade 35% IS THE ONLY GRADE RECOMMENDED FOR INTERNAL USE.

It is used in the production of foods. At this concentration, however, H_2O_2 is a very strong oxidizer and if not diluted, it can be extremely dangerous. It is NOT to be swallowed. 35% H_2O_2 is never to be applied into the mouth without the professional attention of a medical practitioner.

35% Food Grade H_2O_2 must be handled very carefully and diluted properly before use. It will burn the skin—immediate flushing with water is the antidote.

I purchase a 16-ounce bottle of 35% Food Grade Hydrogen Peroxide over the Internet. I then transfer one ounce to a small glass eye-dropper. I store both bottles in the refrigerator freezer to keep them from decomposing. H_2O_2 will not freeze in the freezer. Always use heavy vinyl gloves when handling 35% H_2O_2 to prevent burning the skin.

I dilute my 35% H_2O_2 with distilled water to the appropriate concentration for my needs. I begin with a 2.7% dilution which is a little less than store-bought H_2O_2. I do this by pouring 1 ounce of 35% hydrogen peroxide into a 16-ounce bottle and then adding 12 ounces of distilled water. I also store this in the freezer.

Once I became familiar with H_2O_2, I increased my concentration to 3.5% H_2O_2. This is made by pouring one ounce of 35% H_2O_2 into a 16-ounce bottle and then pouring 11 ounces of distilled water into the bottle. This will be about equal in strength to store-bought H_2O_2.

As I said, this teeth detox is way... way... different. But I, and my entire family, and friends, and business associates, were amazed to see the remarkable results. This teeth detox really DOES work to whiten our chocolate-stained teeth!

And...

We can do it at home... for pennies.

As a family we saved $5600 in dental teeth-whitening bills.

Our teeth and gums are MUCH healthier.

Our entire body is gradually eliminating toxic waste.

Now, all my friends and business associates are whitening their teeth with this detox.

Plus... I'm selling more chocolate products!

and

My Wealth is Increasing!

I'm not sure if this is due to my greater self-confidence because I can whiten my chocolate covered brown teeth stains, or because my business contacts are buying more of my products. I heard that they are spreading the word that they can enjoy super-antioxidant cacao in its many chocolate recipes and forms while still keeping their teeth white.

This safer and more natural teeth detox is spreading world-wide! Now I have a Surprise for you...

SUGAR DOES NOT CAUSE CAVITIES!

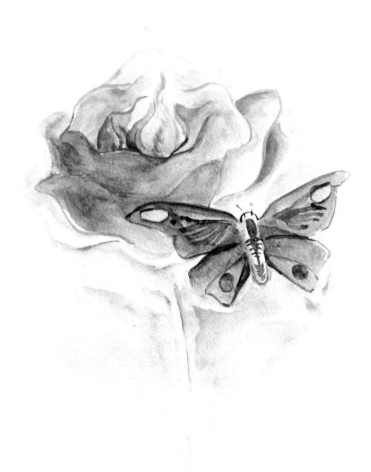

Chapter 23

You'll be SURPRISED to know...

You might ask why, if the teeth detox is a safer and more natural way, do I use man-made beverages like sugared soda colas and chemical solutions like hydrogen peroxide and chlorine bleach?

The problem I see is that as a culture we have made mistakes. We have polluted our environment, abused our bodies, and accumulated toxic waste into our body tissues. As a result we are paying a price with poor health and less joy in our lives. In order to restore our health and well-being we have to detox and eliminate the toxic waste stored in our body tissues. Only then can we enjoy the love of life in as perfect a way as possible; our birthright to a long, generous, and prosperous radiant glow of love in living.

From my research this teeth detox "is" the safest and most natural way to cleanse the teeth of waste. No other system works better, is more convenient, and is less costly. Toxic substances lock tight and hide deep in to the substructure of teeth. They are extremely difficult to clean in a safe and natural way. No other method I'm aware of achieves the same outstanding whitening and detoxing effects as my unique detox. If a better system becomes available, then I will certainly support and promote it, as long as it is effective, safe, and more natural.

Let me explain a few details.

You'll be SURPRISED to know...

Hydrogen Peroxide

Colgate Simply White Night® contains hydrogen peroxide (6.7%). Crest Night Effects® utilizes sodium per-carbonate peroxide (at a concentration of 19%), which is equivalent to 5.3% hydrogen peroxide. Other whiteners on the market have hydrogen peroxide at concentrations up to 17% and more.

My teeth detox gives you complete control over which concentration is best for you and your family. You don't have to buy several different products to find out which one works best with the least side effects such as sensitivity. Plus nothing else is as low-cost, easier to control, and lasts longer.

Phosphoric Acid

Some might question the use of sugared colas with phosphoric acid or citric acid. Actually, my first choice is sparkling white wines, but that would be a problem for young adults who cannot legally purchase alcohol in the United States.

In order to allow hydrogen peroxide to penetrate deeper into the tooth body we have to take advantage of the porous structure of tooth enamel. Acids are the best way to open protein plugs within the enamel tubules. This is the only way I know, at this time, to enter inter-prismatic spaces where chromophores lodge. Sparking white wines are natural and acidic in the range of 3.0pH. Soda colas, although not natural, are a good substitute for those unable to use wine due to age, religious beliefs, or taste.

Organic strawberry juice concentrate has a pH of about 3.0 but it is a little pricey for some compared to colas that are usually on sale. Strawberry juice also has

167

a pinkish color, which will enter the unplugged tubules to further stain the teeth. We do not want this. We need a clear colorless solution with an acidity of about 3.0pH. There are a variety of clear colorless colas at the store that we can choose from to detox teeth. The most effective ones will have phosphoric acid as an ingredient.

Dentist-prescribed bleaching gels usually have potassium hydroxide to help open the pores in enamel. Potassium hydroxide (KOH) has strong degradative properties. It is widely used in the laboratory for the same purposes. Its corrosive properties make it useful as an ingredient in cleaning and disinfecting resistant surfaces and materials. It is often the main active ingredient in chemical "cuticle removers." Potassium hydroxide is also widely used as a way to remove hair from animal hides by leaving the hides in a solution of KOH and water for a few days.

The reason professionally dispensed bleaching gels use potassium hydroxide is just a matter of convenience for packaging, storage, and distribution. Many dentists in the office will pre-treat stubborn stains with 37% phosphoric acid gel. There is nothing better and safer to dissolve and unplug enamel and dentin tubules. The only cheap over-the-counter products at the store to achieve safer, less aggressive, but in a way similar results, are clear colorless soda colas with 3% phosphoric acid. There is a huge difference in safety between 3% and 37%. This is similar to hydrogen peroxide where 37% H_2O_2 is extremely dangerous while 3% is sold at stores for topical application.

Here is another piece of important information. The primary ingredient after water and sugar in many soft drinks is phosphoric acid, which gives the drink its "zing." People usually choose these colas because of their "zing." Yet phosphoric acid is primarily used outside of the soft drink industry as an industrial solvent to clean toilet bowls and to oxidize raw steel so that it can be painted. Is this something you really want to drink or... that your children should be drinking?

I couldn't agree more that one should not drink phosphoric acid. However, industry uses a very high concentration—upwards of 30%. Soda cola has only 3% and is generally recognized as safe to drink in moderation. I recommend rinsing and spitting out only. This is the best way I know to provide easy access with low cost to a home method of opening enamel pores. At this time there is no better, inexpensive, over the counter pretreatment "rinsing" agent to prepare and open the tubules in teeth.

and

as I'd told you...

Sugar Does Not Cause Cavities!

Tooth cavities will be ended simply by rinsing acids off the teeth. ACIDS ALONE, NOT SUGAR, EAT THE ENAMEL. There would be no cavities in the world if all people rinsed acids from their teeth promptly. Using sugared colas with phosphoric acid or citric acid to treat enamel surfaces will cause no permanent harm, as long as we rinse off the solution and re-mineralize the teeth during the detox.

Sodium Hypochlorite (household bleach)

Let's talk a little about sodium hypochlorite (household bleach). At the right concentration it has been used as a disinfectant for over 100 years. It has many of the properties of an ideal anti-microbial agent. At the right concentration it is relatively non-toxic, has no color, and does not stain. It is readily available at low cost. It is lethal to most bacteria, fungi, and viruses. There are no contraindications when it is used as an oral disinfectant.

At low concentrations of 0.1%–0.2% sodium hypochlorite can be used as a debriding and topical antibacterial agent for wounds and skin ulcers. It is used on the battlefield and in hospitals. The American Dental Association Council on Dental Therapeutics proposed using dilute sodium hypochlorite as a topical antiseptic, for irrigation of wounds, and as a mouth rinse.

One of the newest dental rinses on the market, by prescription, is a product called CariFree. It contains Xylitol, Sodium Hydroxide, 0.2% Sodium Hypochlorite, has a 10pH, and is strongly antibacterial and broad spectrum. It is only available from a dentist and has a very high price. You can see that one of the ingredients is 0.2% sodium hypochlorite (diluted household bleach).

I include 0.2% sodium hypochlorite (diluted household bleach) in the teeth detox because sodium hypochlorite rapidly raises the oral environment to about 8.5pH. Re-mineralization occurs more rapidly at pH above 7. It will promote wound healing if you have white spots on your gums from the H_2O_2. Cavities will not form at this high pH, so you should have no concern with the sugar in the cola pre-rinse (in case you do not believe me when I claim sugar does not cause cavities). It is also an excellent antibacterial against gum disease.

You'll be SURPRISED to know...

If you wake up one morning, look into a mirror, stick out your tongue, and see a "Black Tongue" staring you in the face, there is a problem... as you'll learn in my

EPILOGUE...

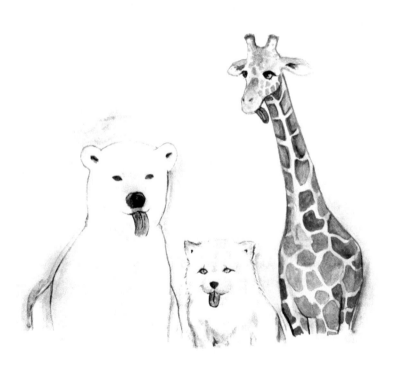

Epilogue

Back Tongue Blues

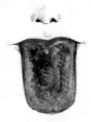

"Look in the mirror—black tongue staring at my face."
These could be lyrics from a song, but if you have a black tongue...

...mission control we have a problem.

Humans do not have black tongues. Humans do not normally wake up with black tongues. A 9th century Tibetan king, Lang Darma, known for his cruelty, had a black tongue. As Buddhists, Tibetans believe in reincarnation, and they feared that this mean king would be reincarnated. Consequently, for centuries Tibetans have greeted one another by sticking out their tongues demonstrating that they do not have black tongues, that they are not guilty of evil deeds, and that they are not incarnations of the malevolent king.

If you wake up with a black tongue, you just might be the Tibetan King, Lang Darma, reincarnated. Good for you!

Buddhists would stick out their tongue as a greeting, because they wanted people to know they were not of a pre-Buddhist religion whose people were supposed to have black tongues. So... pink tongues were stuck out as proof of being Buddhist.

OK, so maybe in an overnight dream you lost your Buddhist faith. A black tongue is your punishment.

Some animals have black tongues. The Chow is a dog with a black tongue. It existed as a hunting dog in China. It was believed in ancient times the dark blue-black mouth and tongue of the Chow Chow, which was exposed when the dog barked, would ward off evil spirits. A few other animals have black tongues, too: the giraffe, polar bear, and several breeds of cattle including the Jersey.

Some dogs will acquire a back tongue due to disease from niacin deficiency. Dogs that suffer from Black Tongue disease will start to lose weight rapidly because they are not eating, as it is painful to them to eat. Niacin, which is also known as Vitamin B3 as well as nicotinic acid, is a water-soluble vitamin, which means that it dissolves in water, and as a result, your pet cannot store it in its body. It must be replenished by your pet's diet, or if necessary, through supplements.

Are you panting and do you have a strange desire to roll over on your back? Look in the mirror again to be sure you didn't die overnight to become reincarnated as a Chow.

While it may be a shocking experience to see a black tongue looking back at you in the mirror, the most common causes of black tongues are not something to become alarmed about. In many cases this is a temporary condition that will go away without any treatment.

Black Hairy Tongue is a medical condition described as a thread-like pattern of dark strands found on the top of your tongue. It looks like your tongue grew a black shag carpet. It is a rather rare condition resulting from overgrowth of bacteria or yeast in your mouth. These bacteria and yeast harbor iron pigments, which give them the black color. The overgrowth of bacteria can also cause cells of the tongue to be shed more slowly, which causes the tongue to take on a hairy appearance.

A black, hairy tongue happens when the papilla on the tongue, normally only one mm in length, grow up to 1.5 cm in length and turn black or brown. This might be harmless, but it looks awful, and is a real possibility occurring most regularly among men who smoke. The condition may also stem from a disturbance in the immune system that allows bacteria to colonize on the tongue. Smoking, especially when combined with poor oral hygiene, certain medicines, and vitamin deficits can lead to the black hairy tongue.

These are the main causes for Black Hairy Tongue:

Antibiotics— may kill "good" bacteria, which control the amount of yeast in your body. An excessive amount of yeast grows and displays itself in your gut, sexual organs, and tongue. It only takes a week of antibiotics to alter the "good" bacteria in your body resulting in overgrowth of yeast. You should always consult your natural health care providers to help you choose the best protection against antibiotic side effects. Usually they will recommend a protocol with prebiotics, probiotics, special foods, and herbs. Once you complete your course of antibiotics, the black tongue should go away on its own. If the black tongue persists, your physician may prescribe an anti-fungal or antibacterial medication for you.

Some asthma inhalers may cause a black tongue in certain individuals. Your physician may want to reduce your dose or switch you to another type of inhaler.

Mineral Supplements— Iron-containing oral solutions used for treatment of iron deficiency anemia cause black stains.

Poor Oral Hygiene— not brushing and/or scraping your tongue might cause an accumulation of bacteria and yeast that may explode into a black colony of fur. Fluids in the mouth contain bacteria and iron pigments (from blood). It is thought that bacteria produce hydrogen sulfide gas as part of their metabolism. This gas reacts with iron in the blood and forms black stain.

Anti-diarrhea medications— bismuth subsalicylate alters the production of bacteria in your mouth and especially on the tongue. Pepto Bismol (and similar over-the-counter medications containing bismuth subsalicylate) is one of the most common causes. This treatment for whatever digestive complaints you may have can also cause your tongue to turn harmlessly black. This is neither harmful nor is the treatment difficult. Simply stop taking the Pepto Bismol. Typically, it will take your tongue about 3 days to return to its normal color.

Smoking— any form of tobacco can contribute to a black tongue. Smoking can alter the chemistry in your mouth, allowing normally harmless bacterial flora to get out of control.

Mouthwashes— Large oral doses of hydrogen peroxide at a 3% concentration may cause irritation and blistering to the mouth. Repeated use of peroxide mouthwashes can alter the amount of bacteria in the mouth.

Caffeinated Beverages— drinking an excessive amount of coffee can change the color of your tongue black.

All these predisposing factors—oral hygiene, smoking, coffee, and mouthwashes—require excessive usage to get a black tongue, and the treatment is simple. Hairy Black Tongue will usually resolve on its own by discontinuing any of the above causative factors and by practicing proper oral hygiene. Tongue brush twice a day and rinse with a diluted hydrogen peroxide mixture of 1 (one) part 3% H_2O_2 and 5 (five) parts water.

IMPORTANT!:
RINSE WITH PLAIN WATER
AFTER USING H_2O_2.

Conditions that cause the immune system to function improperly can also play a role with black tongue discoloration. This is being seen more often in those diagnosed with HIV.

One uncommon but potentially serious disease that can cause black tongue is Sjogren's Syndrome. People with Sjogren's usually have salivary gland dysfunction with xerostomia (dry mouth). The lack of normal salivary function leads to abnormal changes in the bacterial flora of the mouth. This could precipitate a hairy black tongue. If the simpler treatments for black tongue are not effective, your physician may want to evaluate you for this condition.

When you look in the mirror and see a black tongue, ask yourself this question, "Do I feel good, healthy, and strong?" If you are in good health and have a black tongue, then the chances are you are not following my teeth detox protocol. You may have ignored my recommendation to detox for only 2 weeks once you've discovered your safe concentration level. You may have exceeded the suggested dilutions. You may be using a hydrogen peroxide dilution stronger than 3% to rinse with. Any dilution greater than 3% is used only to dab onto your teeth. The bottom line is that if you are not following my teeth detox protocol correctly, you could disrupt the bacterial flora in your mouth. Using excessive quantities of hydrogen peroxide for long periods of time could cause the development of a hairy black tongue. The solution is to stop using hydrogen peroxide and scrape your tongue twice daily.

If the black tongue does not go away and your normal tongue's pink color is not returning, then I strongly suggest you seek professional care from your physician, dentist, and alternative natural health care practitioner.

When I have a question about the way I look or feel, I always visit my Oriental Medical Acupuncturist before visiting my Western Medical Doctor. Certainly, if I'm in need of urgent trauma care due to a major accident I'll run straight to the nearest medical emergency clinic. If I'm suffering from ruptured, crushed, broken, burnt, slashed, torn, gouged, chipped, cracked, or dislocated body parts, then I'm definitely first in line at the 'Doc in the Box'. But if I'm not feeling well and my heart is still beating, lungs breathing, and eyes, nose, ears still attached to my head, then I believe it is best to make

the earliest appointment with a Master Herbal Acupuncturist or Ayurvedic practitioner. I'm convinced
an alternative health care practitioner with thousands
of hours of education in the prevention and long term
care of energetic imbalances is by far my better choice.
These are the professionals best trained to guide me to
my goal of being as happy, youthful, and energetic at
age 125 years as I'm sure I'll be at 75... actively mountain biking, skiing, and practicing vigorous martial arts.

The following interesting story proves my point.
Please understand that they didn't teach me alternative
health care in dental school, and I am in no way quali-
fied to discuss the topic. I can only relate to you what
my friend, Kim Blankenship, L.Ac. has to say about the
topic of Black Tongue.

At one time I had strained an area of rib cage car-
tilage, and an herbal formula teapill was prescribed to
support the healing process. I can't say who invented
the teapill, but my best understanding is that in ancient
times herbs were initially foraged in the wild, cut to size,
dried, and then prepared by simmering the cut pieces
in hot water. Later in the history of time the dried cut
herbs were ground into a powders, carried in pouches,
and... as needed, a hot tea was brewed to drink.

In more modern days the powders were formed into
a dough ball from a concentrated paste. The dough is
rolled out and machine cut into small round pieces that
are then spun into quality teapills. In the final stage, a
tiny amount of talcum (hua shi) and activated carbon
are added for smoothness. The teapills are coated with a
fine layer of botanical wax to provide for easier swallowing and to help naturally preserve freshness. In this way
the teapill herbal formula could be swallowed directly,

which is more convenient than, for example, brewing tea during your lunch break at a local fast food diner.

These teapills were a novelty for me, and after taking them for a day I would look in the mirror, and observe... staring straight at me was... a Black Tongue! I had no idea what was the cause of the Black Tongue, because, as I said, dental schools usually don't teach alternative medicine. After a little research I discovered that it was the "activated carbon" in the coating that imparted a temporary Black Tongue. Once I finished the remedy... over a specific time period... my tongue returned to its normal pink color. I did, however, have many comedic moments sticking my Black Tongue out at friends and fellow workers.

I decided to contact Kim Blankenship, L.Ac., and ask him more questions about Black Tongue as it related to Chinese medicine. Here are bits and pieces of our conversation:

LS... Kim Blankenship, would you please define Black Tongue coating as interpreted by traditional Oriental Medicine.

KB... Black Tongue Coating in Chinese Medicine
The tongue is a valuable diagnostic tool in Chinese Medicine, a real-time display of the state of various organ systems that is typically used in conjunction with pulse diagnosis to give the acupuncturist or herbalist a complete picture of the patient's current condition. Practitioners can discern which organ systems may be in a weakened or excited state, whether the body's Yin and Yang are in balance, and a world of other information revealing the condition of the body's physical and energetic internal landscape.

A black tongue coating is fortunately seldom seen in clinic. The two possible causes for a black tongue coating in Chinese medicine are polar opposites of each other and both indicative of temperature extremes within the body. A black tongue coating that is dry and cracked reveals extreme heat while a black coating that is wet indicates extreme cold. In either case, immediate treatment is warranted. On the one hand, acupuncture to clear heat in concert with a cooling herbal formula is necessary, and on the other hand warming herbs and moxibustion are required to bring the body back into balance.

Kim Blankenship, L.Ac.

LS... What do you mean when you say it is "fortunately seldom seen in clinic"?

KB... It is "fortunately seldom seen" because it is only seen with extreme conditions and most people would have hopefully already received treatment before reaching such an extreme.

LS... Where is Black Tongue coating seen?

KB... Most likely in patients with a very high fever or extremely low body temperature of long duration.

LS... Have you ever seen it?

KB... No. I've seen a dark brown coating that possibly could have progressed to black if the patient had gone untreated.

LS... What are the odds that this type of extreme would walk into a dentist office for a diagnosis?

KB... Slight. People in that condition would not likely be seeking dental care at that time.

LS... Could a person in this condition drive himself to the dentist?
KB... Possibly, but I don't think that would be a priority.

LS... More often related to an age group?
KB... Not necessarily.

LS... Could swine flu bring one to this condition?
KB... I doubt it based on the information that is currently available on the new strain.

LS... What would be some of the 'obvious' western medicine symptoms associated with these extremes?
KB... High fever or low body temperature.

LS... What are the odds of recovering back to a normal pink tongue?
KB... A lot would depend on the age and constitution of the patient, but I would think recovery would be possible.

If you have more questions for Kim Blankenship, L.Ac. you can email him at Jadespirit@mac.com

After our brief conversation I breathed a sigh of relief knowing that a person with this type of Black Tongue coating would not normally be seeking dental care. If, however, someone in this dire condition did somehow drive to my office for help, I would immediately refer him to his medical doctor, even though in my heart I believe it would be better to first see an alternative medical practitioner. This 'standard referral' protects my assets against a possible malpractice judgment. I would then suggest that the patient also see an alternative health care practitioner such as an Oriental Medical Doctor or an Ayurvedic practitioner.

You must understand that dentists are under extreme pressure from the "health police", a.k.a. the Western medical authorities and their lawyers. We must always, first always, and ultimately always refer to a Western trained medical doctor for diseases not related to the oral cavity. If we do not follow this protocol, then the "health police" will come breaking down our doors to file claims against our professional practice. All this to retain control of the medical 'business' of doctoring and keep their fingers tightly wound around the financial dollars of the consumer.

Let me be perfectly clear. This book, *The Teeth Whitening Cure*, was written with one purpose in mind—to be a primer to help you tailor your own personal medical and dental health insurance plan. If you plan on living a healthy, vibrant 125 years… and more, then you must insure and protect yourself from big-money dental products manufacturing interests. Some of the biggest profit makers for these money-hungry giant corporations include teeth whitening kits.

Sadly, I have to admit that many dentists feed into this cash generating, teeth bleaching machine. Admittedly, until recently my dental practice was one of them, though not anywhere near to the extreme which seems lately to be all too common. In fact, some profit-obsessed dentists are even using subliminal messages trying to convince patients that their teeth should be whiter... falling victims to big corporate media manipulation when the powers that be, greedy mega-corporations, illustrate the huge profits available to them from teeth whitening.

Believe me I'm not saying that teeth whitening is completely unnecessary. But if your dentist or dental hygienist hounds you to have your teeth bleached to improve your smile, then you can be sure their heavy-handed push is making somebody rich.

Fortunately I have discovered a way to whiten teeth with your health first in mind. I now understand that there is a safer and healthier way to whiten teeth. This new way of thinking about teeth whitening takes advantage of the body's innate ability to detoxify itself of harmful substances found naturally within the body and also absorbed from the outside environment. And... you can do this right in the comfort of your home, at a tremendous cost savings.

Ancient Chinese, Tibetan, and Indian medicine from at least 10,000 years ago had well documented the connection between dental health and whole-body health. Hippocrates (ca. 400 BC), the father of Western medicine, treated arthritis by pulling infected teeth. Today researchers are discovering and investigating new links between an unhealthy mouth and serious whole body health problems. Western medicine has scientifically proven that at least 90% all systemic diseases produce oral signs and symptoms.

The health of your mouth generally reflects the health of your entire body. At any given time there are more than 500 species of bacteria in your mouth.

These bacteria form living, conscious colonies, which fluctuate, balance, and communicate with themselves and every other cell of your body. According to ancient records of philosophy, mathematics, and medicine this cellular communication is called the 'dance of life'.

After reading the valuable information in this book you can now lighten and whiten your teeth, protect your smile, and improve overall body health. Teeth whitening can be done in a smarter, safer, and healthier way, if you keep my teeth detox in mind.

Lester J. Sawicki, D.D.S.

HYPERLINK "http://www.RevolutionTooth.com/"
http://www.RevolutionTooth.com/

Printed in the USA
CPSIA information can be obtained
at www.ICGtesting.com
LVHW021610010524
779048LV00010B/394